Camille Pablo Russell
The Path of the Buffalo
Medicine Wheel

I dedicate this book to my children:
Layne, Autumn, Jerred, Charlie, Raphael and Noah.
Grandchildren: Kaylie, Willie, Illiana, Penelope, Darrian, Jordan,
Huge Jordan and Alex Ried and to the rest of my family and
extended family through Canada, Europe, and to all mankind
in the hopes of a better future for all.

Camille Pablo Russell

Fifth Edition

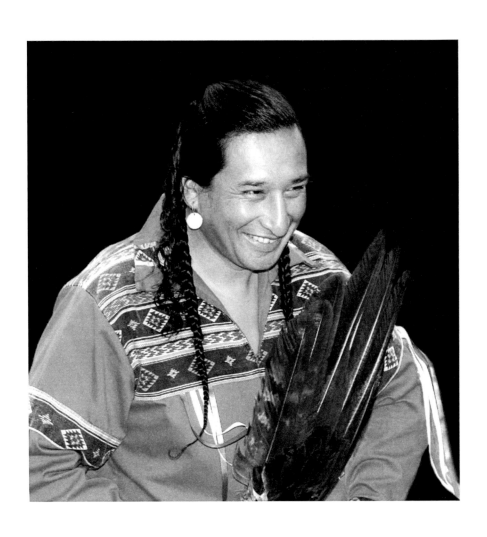

Camille Pablo Russell
The Path of the Buffalo
Medicine Wheel

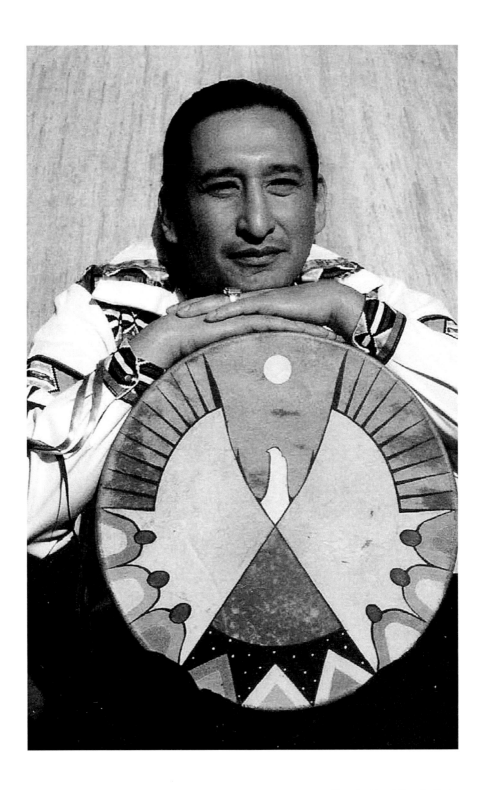

The Path of the Buffalo

Contents

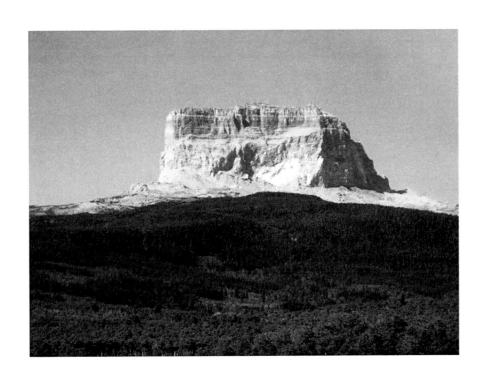

The Path of the Buffalo

Foreword

Pablo has the key to open hearts during his lectures and workshops, and to help us understand the essence of his teachings. Pablo is endowed with the ability to touch and understand a human being on a personal level. There is a deeper holistic connection to all beings, to the great mystery, like old memories, when we pray and sing and celebrate the ancient ceremonies that continuously sustain the balance of nature, life, wisdom and serenity.

I have attended many of Pablo's seminars over the last years, and each time I find new insights helping me along the circle of life of my personal Medicine Wheel.

There are countless books on the Native American Medicine Wheel, and you may wonder why this one differs from all the other books.

This is an absolutely unique and exceptional transcript, based on ancient traditions of the Blackfoot Native Americans. These teachings have now, for the first time in history, been recorded in writing. In order to stay as close to the original traditions as possible, as well as respecting the teachings of the Elders, this transcript was written according to the chronology, context, and structure of Pablo's workshops and seminars.

This book offers the reader not only a great opportunity to grasp the spirit Chief Mountain of Pablo, but also the spirit of his lectures and teachings. As well as learn-ing about your own behavioral patterns, and how to explain and deal with them, you will also to learn about the deep connection between the native culture and spirituality.

Martina Moser

I have in this book continuously supported the Wheels with different examples on the following topics: mother, grandparents, dad, society, mentors, and vision quests.

Camille Pablo Russell

Introduction

My name is Camille Pablo Russell. My Native American name is "Shooting in the Air". Born on the Blood Reserve in Southern Alberta, I grew up very close to my grandparents, and learned a lot about my roots and traditions. Over the past 20 years, I have lectured in Europe on Mental Health, Coaching, Traditional Herbs and Leadership Management. I was invited to several Esoteric Conferences. I am working in Calgary, Alberta at the Elbow River Healing Lodge as spiritual counselor and as native coordinator at the local Correctional Institution.

My workshops are based on the principle of "Follow the Buffalo". To native people the buffalo represents the qualities of perseverance, facing the storms of life and walking into them.

At the age of 19, I started preparing for sun dancing, and my learning continued for eleven years. Then, I was granted the role of leader in the Sundance. I continued to learn from the Sundance leaders about the "warrior ways", as well as the "way of the holy pipe". These teachings are the foundation for understanding the four parts of a human being and ways of centering.

My leader followed our oral tradition in teaching the medicine wheel, but he put this knowledge onto a diagram, to support teaching the principles to modern thinking people.

After learning for 13 years I was granted the right to teach on my own. My workshops are based on this, and other tools, which have helped many people to see things, they have to correct, and take new directions, not only in their lives, but in their work, and to take the steps necessary to improve their quality of life.

This book is a transcript of the spoken word contents of my lectures and workshops of the "Path of the Buffalo". As I have already mentioned, I grew up with my grandparents listening to stories and teachings, which were passed on orally by our elders to the next generations. For the Blackfoot Nation, as well as many indigenous people, it was only a puddle jump from the old days of oral tradition to urban life and virtual media. Our native Blackfoot language has rarely been written down or printed in books. My first book is transcribed from my mother tongue captured on a recorder.

The Medicine Wheel

First Diagram

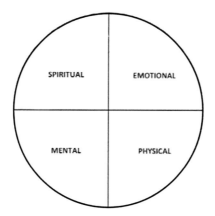

Second Diagram

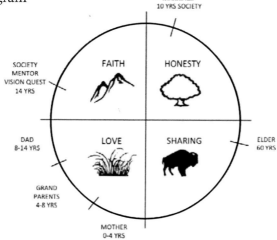

Third Diagram

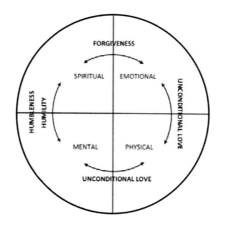

The Medicine Wheel

First of all I want to express my views on the medicine wheel. There are a lot of medicine wheels out there. People put labels on their medicine wheels and certify them these, days but, I always wonder who certifies these medicine wheels. I guess the only one who could certify the medicine wheel, is the one who came up with the wheel them self.

A medicine wheel in my understanding – from my teacher – is a diagram illustrating or supporting a native philosophy or teaching.

In the past these teachings were not put into a diagram. They were just orally told to an individual by a person, who knew the proper way of living, and what it took to do that. The medicine wheel is a very current thing. In the distant past, medicine wheels where not drawn on buffalo robes, and people did not sit in front of these buffalo robes, which hung on a tripod. The elder did not have a stick pointing to the drawing of the medicine wheel and then explaining it. In those days the elders talked and the student imagined what he was trying to talk about, and understood in that way.

Today it is a modern time and a lot of people do not live for the moment. A lot of memories are put into reading and writing and this is what the mind frame has become for everyone, including aboriginal people. So to explain a native teaching or philosophy or way of being people started making diagrams. As native people we think in a circle, so naturally our drawing is going to be a circle and then within this circle is an explanation, a teaching. So the name for this teaching became a 'medicine wheel'.

There are many different types of medicine wheels, because there are many different kinds of teachings. Different tribes explain the teachings in different ways, with different animals etc. Some medicine wheels will have colors and directions. Others will have animals and plants to explain a teaching.

Today we don't think the way people used to think. There are a lot of things that are lacking from our ability to understand the old way of teaching. The sense of dreams and following your dreams has been restricted due to norms and stopping of natural growth, and all these restrictions that people put on children today. Adults don't allow children to believe and connect naturally anymore. Adults put a set of norms and expectations on a child at a very early age, which stops their imagination skills. Children start to compete with the rest of society, at a very young age.

When children are old enough to think for themselves, it is hard for them to imagine and understand fully what the elders are trying to teach them. In order to help the new generation understand these old teachings, we have to adapt the teaching skills to this new generation. So we draw circles, divide them into four sections, and we hang the diagram on the wall.

Some wheels have colors in them, seasons, animals and directions. This is just to explain what the teacher is trying to teach them. There is not one true medicine wheel, nor is there one way a medicine wheels should be. There are many different kinds of medicine wheels out there, trying to explain a philosophy or a way of life, that belonged to the people of North America.

There are many different teachings and many different types of wheels. They come from native teachings from our elders, and the medicine wheel that I am talking about here, was taught to me from my teacher. He taught me and gave me the rights to use it to help people.

This medicine wheel that I am talking about, is the explanation of my teacher. This is the one that he taught me and that I had to live by, learn by and to change my ways by, in order for me to be able to share it with other people.

It took 13 years of sitting beside my teacher, being his apprentice, serving him tea, watching him doing this wheel diagram for audiences over and over again for me to learn the ways. And just when I thought I knew the wheel, something else popped up that I didn't understand or see or realize or discover, and it continued and continued. Along the way I applied some of those teachings to my personal life and grew and learned and healed from it – not saying that I am perfect – but it did help me change my view on life. It helped me open up my heart and discover who I am as a human being on this earth, and also as a son to my people.

One day my leader said: "Okay now you get up to the board and you talk about the medicine wheel". Of course I was shocked because the anticipation of teaching the wheel had long gone from my ego, because all I did was sit and observe him for 13 years, so I never thought that I would teach it. Then finally he said: "okay you teach it!" So I got up and explained the wheel to the best of my ability at that time.

He critiqued me and said that I did a good job. Later, when we were alone, I questioned him and asked him why he asked me to do the wheel – now – 13 years later. He laughed and he said: "It is very simple, son. You had to fix your wheel first before you can teach it."

That left a very significant realization inside of me. That you first have to heal and understand what you are teaching and go through it yourself before you can turn around and try to teach or share it with others.

There is a saying that the best teachers are people who are going through it themselves.

Heal yourself before helping others

What I find today in a lot of cases in the world is that people study to be of service to people, but they themselves have not healed the things they preach. In some cases the people who are in the helping field have personal problems themselves. You see this in professions like nursing, teaching, psychiatry, clergy or social work. You realize that in many cases they did not deal with their problems on a personal level.

To compensate for that, they get an education and they try to help people with the same problems, which creates what some people call a shadow or the dark side of themselves.

Probably these people are not aware of this mechanism when they go through it, but perhaps they become aware of it later on in life.

They do not have the elders, and the mentors that talked with them about these things and teach them about behaviors of people. When I was growing up, I was given examples of different lifestyles, and why that was that way or why that person was like that. They would give you an understanding if you follow this road this could happen, and if you go that way that could happen. So you are not aware, because there is no one around teaching you behaviors of people, or even telling you about your behavior.

If an elder in our culture sees somebody becoming a professional caregiver without dealing with his or her own problems first, then the elder would tell you that you should fix yourself first, before you consider helping people. That is the traditional way. So the person knows it in advance and starts working on her or himself before she / he becomes a professional caregiver. This is what the elders would teach. This is the problem with society today, that there are no elders to talk to, or no connections to the elders in the society. So these insights are not being shared or taught so that people become aware of it.

This is where this diagram comes from, and the teachings, which is a Blackfoot concept of life. But it applies to any lifestyle of any tribe or any nationality, because it is about the human being. So anybody could relate to this wheel and use it and it, has been used for thousands of years. The wheel is still valid today, and people still need the wheel to fix their life, because we do not have the traditional lifestyle, we used to have.

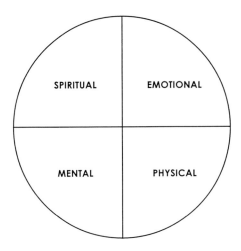

The first diagram is about the spiritual, emotional, physical and mental, which is a human being. Each one of us has these four parts that make us who we are – a human being, an individual. We all have a spiritual part we all have a mental part we all have an emotional part and that is all encased in a physical body.

All these four parts need to have some attention in each of them, and when there is more attention in some areas, and less in another, then you are not centered, and things are not going the way they should be going in your life. So what you try to do, is to see where you are in each section.

When I am talking about spirituality, in the realm of spirituality, I am talking about when you talk to the Creator. Not meditation or yoga or other things like that. I am talking about you having a conversation with your higher power the Creator or God, where you are asking for things, or giving thanks for things on a regular basis. If you include Him in your life, then He becomes a part of you, your friend. Not to be feared, but to be your maker. You should be comfortable in talking to Him. Not only asking for things, but also giving thanks for the good things as well as the bad things. Through this spiritual part, what develops is the ability to forgive. We learn to forgive ourselves, forgive others and forgive ourselves for hurting others. That is what we learn in spirituality, when we talk to the Creator every day.

You also develop the awareness, of being able to put yourself in another person's shoes. So you can feel how it is to be in another person's shoes, when you are behaving a certain way which can make you change your behavior immediately to have some self-control, self-discipline or maybe rewording what you are about to express.

You evaluate yourself and you ask yourself, how much time do I spend talking to the Creator? Asking for things, giving thanks to Him for things strengthening my faith and understanding His teachings, trying to practice them and being aware of the Creator. How much time do I devote in this area? Some people devote a lot of time, some a little bit of time and others do not really think about it.

People have a different awareness of spirituality. So what you do is that you make an arch from one point to another, to indicate how much time you spend in there: a little bit, or maybe a lot. So you see for yourself where you are in that section, and draw it on the wheel.

Then you go down to the mental, which is comprised of two types of ego: The positive ego and the negative ego. The positive ego is the part of your brain that says: you are good, you can do it, you know what you are doing, you are confident, you can fix this and you can make it. Then there is the negative part that says: poor me, do it for me, take care of me, help me, pity me, feel sorry for me. So we have both of these parts. On an average day you want to try to see for yourself, which one is stronger or more prominent in your thinking. Is it the positive or is it the negative one? Special days or hard days are not what I am talking about. If you won an award of course the positive will be higher. If you are sick or lost a loved one, then the negative will be higher. On an average day which one is higher? If the positive is higher then you draw a bigger arch. If the negative is bigger then draw a smaller arch.

Then you go to the emotional and then you find out with yourself: can I express my feelings, am I afraid to express my feelings, do I know what I am crying about, can I say I love you, can I hug. Then you draw a bigger arch. But if your heart is closed, and you have a hard time expressing your feelings or hugging or accepting or giving love, or if you are crying, but you do not know why you are crying, and you do not understand your feelings, then you draw a smaller arch.

Then we go to the physical. It is pretty straight forward. If you eat right, you feel healthy, you exercise regularly, then you draw a big arch. If you do not really watch what you eat and do not really exercise, then you draw a smaller arch. If you are ill and for instance you have rheumatism or diabetes or heart problems, then you draw a smaller arch.

Now you can see that the wheel is not all the same. It is not centered. Then you wonder how it came to be like this. What happened in my life for things to become like this? Which patterns have I acquired or made for myself for this to occur, and then you go to the next wheel, which is another diagram which is the journey of an individual from birth to death and everything in between.

This medicine wheel, is just to give you an example what it could look like. Now it's your turn for self-evaluation, how to draw your own wheel.

Examples of Smaller and Bigger Arches:

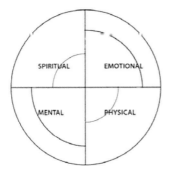 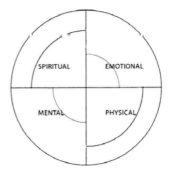

Weak in Physical and Spiritual   Weak in Mental and Emotional
Strong in Mental and Emotional   Strong in Physical and Spiritual

Self-Evaluation - How to Draw Your Own Wheel

How much energy do I spend in each area? Then you go on explaining the size of the arch in each section.

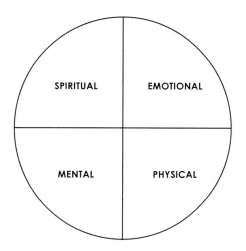

Spiritual

In the spiritual you ask yourself the following questions:

How much time do you spend talking to God or the Creator? Do you follow the teachings that you were brought up with daily? Do you feel secure in your beliefs? Do you practice or know rituals or ceremonies? Do you ask for help? Do you give thanks?

These are the things you ask yourself when you are evaluating your spiritual area.

Mental

Mental is made up of positive and negative ego:

Positive ego: I can do it, the cup is half full, look on the I can agree. Negative ego: poor me, take care of me, do it for me, feel sorry for me, no I cannot work with you. So these are the positive and negative sides of the mental part.

If you are thinking in a positive way then you draw the arch in the mental area bigger. And the more positive you think the bigger the arch.

Emotional

To see how big the arch in the emotional area is you ask yourself the following questions:

Is your heart open? Can you express your feelings? Do you know why you are crying? Can you give and receive love? Are you happy?

These are the things you can ask yourself to determine how big you draw the arch in the emotional area.

Physical

Physical: Do you exercise? Do you eat right? Are you happy with your body? Do you get enough rest and sleep? Do you feel well?

So, that is the first diagram, which explains the arches. You use these questions to evaluate yourself in each area and draw your wheel. Then you see in which areas you are stronger and in which areas you need more energy.

Spirituality

The keywords for spirituality are: connection to the soul, purpose in life, support, love, compassion, sharing and kindness. Spirituality supports ownership of feelings; it supports care for Mother Earth and animals, plants, water and rocks. Your belief in a higher power influences right choices. Also support, faith and trust are established through spirituality.

These are the things you are taught, and these are the things that happen inside of you when you are dealing with spirituality.

These things come from the emotional but when you have spiritual teachings it helps you to be kind and have compassion. You already have those feelings, but spirituality tells you how to use them in different situations.

Example:
Just like a little child, he knows naturally how to share. He never went to church and he does not know about God, but he has this emotion of sharing and not sharing. Then he goes to church with his mom and dad, and he hears the preacher say, that when you share you are in God's good books. So now he knows. He already knew how to share naturally before he went to church; he knew how to laugh naturally; be happy naturally; to hug; give love and get love naturally. He got those from mom and dad, but when he was introduced into spirituality, they were teaching him how to love God; how to love mom and dad, and he learned that it is a good thing to love all people. So spirituality is showing you how to place each emotion.

This is what spirituality is. Showing you how to feel in a positive way whether it is love, anger, jealousy or compassion. Spirituality tells you how to cope with that feeling and express it in a healthy way. So this is what spirituality is doing in addition to talking to God and finding your purpose in life.

It is supporting the emotional by educating it according to God's laws.

Example:
A kid could be in the woods and break flowers or whatever. But later he is taught that these are your relatives, it is nature and your spirits and plants and rocks. Now the kid is not going back to rip the flowers down. He knows now that there is a spirit in them, so it creates respect and it

creates a relationship
with nature, which disciplines that person to think in a healthier way towards the environment. So this is what spirituality is doing.

The Mind

The mind makes the body function with its physical features; it controls spiritual beliefs, emotional expression and it judges the body. So the mental controls your spiritual beliefs and it controls your emotional expression.

Maybe you want to hug somebody, but your mind will say: "no, that is not appropriate" or "that is not right" or "you might get hurt" or "they might get the wrong impression".

Your mind will stop you from hugging. It controls your emotion.
Example:
If you are in the train and you want to get mad and yell at someone and there is a bunch of people around, then maybe the brain says: "this is not a good time to do that".

So the mind is controlling your expression and your feelings. And your mind judges the body. Every time you look in the mirror you judge your body – positively or negatively. Maybe you think you look great or maybe you think you should lose weight. The mind will try to help you survive. It has survival instincts.

Example:
If there was a fire or a wild animal close by then you will not just stand there. You will run away. You will try to save yourself. You are not sitting there, thinking it out and discussing if you should do this or that. If you see a car coming towards you then you will jump out of the way without thinking or discussing or feeling.

That is what the brain does. It's got survival instincts. It is created for you to survive in different situations. The brain sets the impulse to shoot out adrenalin, so you can run away or save yourself in other ways.

Then the other function of the brain is to maintain interest. The chemicals in the brain create this interest. It releases things to make you curious. It releases things so you can have vitality like happiness, excitement, joy and sexual desires. Your brain is introducing these chemicals into your body. There are stress relievers in there supposedly. If you had a non-stressed mom then you should have stress-relieving endorphins in you – also for pain. So the brain is creating its own painkiller. So you are not hurt. That painkiller goes to your physical pain as well as your emotional pain.

So this is what your brain is doing.

The negative sides of the brain are that it is judgmental, insecure, lazy, selfish, self-destructive, sabotaging, it is afraid of rejection; it wants the easy way out and the most important thing is, that it does not accept its shadow or its dark sides.

The positive abilities of the brain are that it supports determination; it is problem solving; it has faith; it makes decisions and it is a logical thinker. It does logical thinking as opposed to the heart, which is not doing that.

Example:
If you are not expressing your emotions in a healthy way or have borders:

Let us say that one day your heart runs away with you and you fall in love with someone who lives in Australia. He asks you to come home with him and your heart says: "yes, let us go!" Then your mind will interrupt and it says: "wait a minute!" "How are you going to live and support yourself?" and "You have all these things to consider". So instead of just going where your heart wants to go, your brain will make you think realistically about it. Your mind is telling your heart "wait a minute, let us consider this!" If it were just left up to your emotions then you would just go and maybe you would not know how to get back home, or did not have enough money to come back home if it did not work out. Or maybe it works out and you have a great life.

For most people, the logical part of your mind overrules the emotional part too much.

Emotional

The emotional side of you: It is heart feelings like being happy, angry, sad, lonely, content, share, compassion, forgiveness, kindness, love. Then the physical attributes of the heart is that it moves blood through the body; it is a connection to the soul; it accepts the dark sides of you; it influences the mind; it has heart feelings and desires. So the emotional part influences the mind and it has desires.

Physical

Your physical body is the image of mother earth.

Your body is a shell for your soul. So your spirit is inside your body, which is the shell. It makes your soul go through life and find your purpose and have children. Without your soul your body does not function and when you die your soul leaves your body. It does not stay in the body. When you die your body dies and decays. There will be no more of you. That is why I am saying that your body is a shell for your soul. Your body is here to fulfill your purpose in life.

Example:
You are born and then all of a sudden you became crippled and you could not walk so you had a wheel chair.

Before the accident you were walking around maybe you are an athlete, you climb mountains and you are really selfish, you are really in good shape and you think you are it. Everybody desires you.

Then you have an accident. You cannot walk and you become humble and you have humility. Then you change your attitude and you find that you have to work for people and help people in some way.

So through all this pain and suffering you find your purpose in life, which is to work from the wheel chair whether it is making books or talking. So in that person's life, he had to break his back or whatever for his purpose in life to be revealed to him. So that is what I am talking about when I say that your body or your shell is here to fulfill your purpose in life.

Example:
If you are going to Sundance you need a body that is prepared for sun dancing. Or maybe you had a heart condition and you got out of it because of sun dancing.

Your body is designed to go through an experience to reveal your purpose in life whatever your purpose is.

Example:
Maybe you are very beautiful and you live in a little town. Then you go to the city and some model agency guy takes your picture. Now you are a model, you live in the city, you are making money, and you are sending money to your family. Your body is supposed to help you with what you are supposed to go through. Or maybe you are a craftsman or a farmer so you need to have a certain type of body to be able to do that.

The body characteristics and how they work:

You have blond hair and blue eyes: you are Scandinavian. So your body is revealing to whomever that you are from Scandinavian descend. Or you have brown eyes and black hair with braids. A person when they look at you will see that this human being is a North American Indian by his features: black hair, high cheek bones, chief mountain nose, that person is a native. Or a person has curly hair and really dark skin and big lips: he is from Africa. Or a short guy with slit eyes: he is from Asia.

Your body characteristics are identifying you to the world. It is like a plant. Its appearance is showing the world what it is. This is Daisy; this is Juniper and that is Sweet Pine. That is what your body also does. It is showing your characteristics and nationality. And those characteristics are affected by feelings, thoughts and environment.

If you are sad or depressed then you are either not eating at all or eating a lot. Or if you are thinking too much or on the go all the time, you cannot sleep or do not get enough sleep. Those things will affect your body and so will the environment. If you live in a smog city then you are going to have a poor health condition compared to someone living in the mountains with fresh air. So your body is affected by your thinking; it is affected by what you are feeling; by your environment and by what you eat of course, which is part of the environment.

The physical does what your heart and mind want it to do. Whatever your mind says your body will do it. Or whatever your heart says your body will do.

Example:
So if you care about somebody or are married to somebody then you will take your clothes off and have sex. But if you do not know this stranger and you have never seen him before then your mind and heart says to

your body "No, you are not going to have sex with him – you do not know him."

Your body on its own wants whatever: eat, have sex or go to the bathroom. It does what it needs to do. It has no shame or guilt. If you ate human meat your body will digest it. But your mind and your heart will say: "gross, this is human meat!" and then your body will throw up because your mind is rejecting it. It does what the mind and heart wants. So this is what the body is doing. And it is a tool for the Creator.

Example:
So an artist will start painting, and the Creator goes through the artist and he paints a great picture. Or the medicine man is doctoring, and the spirits and the Creator go through the medicine man and doctor the person. So it is being used as a tool for the Creator as well.

The Bridges of the Medicine Wheel

Now we go to the bridges, how to transfer energy from one section to the next section:

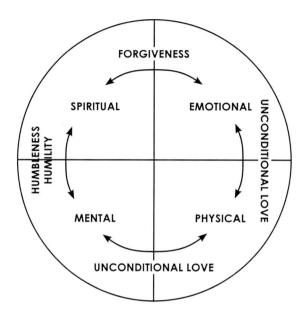

To transfer energy from spiritual to emotional or vice versa the bridge is called forgiveness.

Steps to proper forgiveness:
In the first wheel when you evaluate yourself, and you see how much energy you put into each section, some will be bigger than others. What you need to do, is to give some energy from the ones where you have more attention in, and feed the ones that you have less attention in, and there needs to be a bridge that connects the two.

Spiritually to emotionally:
If you are strong spiritually and you are weak emotionally and you want to give more energy to emotion or vice versa, then the bridge that connects this energy to pass back and forth is called forgiveness.

Forgiveness Has Three Steps That Makes it True Forgiveness.

First you have to understand the story behind the situation, that got you hurt - perhaps with your parents, and the story behind their behavior towards you. Once you understand that story and hear all of it perhaps you will realize, that they grew up the same way as you did. They may lack parenting skills or affection or whatever, and this is the reason for their behavior.

Now you understand why they did what they did. Then the next step is to accept the fact that this is how they are, and this is what they have, and to accept them just as they are and not to be resentful. What follows after this is true forgiveness. You forgive from the head and the heart, and you get a better relationship with them. This is true forgiveness.

If it is from emotional to physical then you must love yourself unconditionally so you accept your body for the way it is, you accept your sexuality, and you are open to feel like a different person. You are open to feel who you are and be okay with loving yourself and be okay with thinking that you are a special person and just accepting yourself unconditionally the way you are. And then from physical to mental, or mental to physical it is the same thing: Unconditional love.

To accept your looks the way they are, to accept your body type the way it is, to accept your voice, your hair color, your height, your nose, your ears, your eyes., to accept yourself unconditionally the way you are; these are the bridges to giving energy back and forth.

And then from mental to spiritual or spiritual to mental, the bridge is called humbleness and humility, and this is to suppress the ego so you are teachable, and you are able to listen and to learn instead of being a 'know it all'. You have to get past that ego part of yourself and you go through ceremonies to learn humbleness and humility. Then you are open to receive the messages from the Creator, or from the teacher about Creator and about spirituality. This is what you develop in spirituality from the mental or from connecting the two into giving energy. It is called humbleness and humility.

Wanting and Needing

There is a big difference between wanting and needing. Sometimes we overlook the things we need because of the things that we want. Let's say you want a million dollars, but what you need to pay bills is not that much.

You need to love yourself, you need healing, you need awareness, you need family, you need love, you need to give love, you need to express love, you need love to be expressed to you, you need to forgive and people need to forgive you, you need a job, you need to eat, you need a home, you need transportation, you need goals and you need a purpose in life.

There are things you need to survive as an individual: clothing, hygiene. To survive in a good way. You need to have hobbies and to keep busy and to keep things balanced in your life. You need to know your roots, you need to know the history of your people and your linage, you need to live for the moment more often, you need to share, you need to be kind, you need to understand, you need to be strong, you need to overcome your fears, you need to overcome laziness. At times you need to overcome depression or sadness, you need to be aware of nature and the cycle of life. These are the things that a human being needs to have a good healthy life.

What you want is a million dollars, the prettiest partner you can get, the prettiest body you can get. You want perfection but you do not want to work on yourself to get that perfection. In order for that perfection to occur it has to mirror perfection.

Sometimes a person is beautiful in appearance, but inside they are not beautiful so they do not get what they want, they just get the opposite person or maybe somebody like themselves, who is nice on the outside but not on the inside.

And even though they are together, they seek this purity within themselves and what they need, they do not appreciate or respect, or maybe they are not aware that they need these things.

Sometimes you want the prettiest girl in the world to be with you and maybe there is a person who is maybe not the prettiest, but she is pretty and she cares for you, and has the love for you, but yet you want something even better than that.

We are never satisfied with what is in front of us, or could be in front of us, because we want more than what we deserve, or what we earned or who we are. In order for us to get something more than what we are, we need to change to be more than what we are. Then we can get something more. We want things that are not attainable sometimes, but what we need is something that is very important to have. What we want would be nice to have, or ideal to have, but what we need is more important than what we want. So we ask Creator to help us to get what we need, but what we want we try to go get it ourselves, by working harder and setting goals to get it.

Why is it Important to Live for the Moment?

Living for the moment allows your mind and heart to shake hands and agree. Most often times our heart says one thing and our mind says another, and they often disagree with each other. Therefore there is a conflict and usually the head wins the conflict, and the heart does not, and then you make the wrong choices and the repercussions come back to you and you feel bad about it. The consequences make you feel bad about your first choice. So what you want to do, is to make the right choice, which is when the heart and mind agree.

So in order for them to agree, you must do something that makes you live for the moment. Some things that make you live for the moment are hobbies or things of interests like fishing or archery, sports, bird watching or sewing or beading. Every individual has different interests that make them happy and lose track of time. They are so into what they are doing, that when they become aware of reality again, two or three hours, have gone by unnoticed, but there has been a healing within themselves and their mind, and their heart are friendlier towards each other, and decisions are easier to make.

Hobbies and things of interest create living for the moment, and then there is the other, which is the spiritual and physical done together at the same time. When you take something physical and spiritual in combination with each other, then you also create this living for the moment, which creates peace in the mind, and peace in the heart and forgiveness starts to occur. Loving yourself, awareness of the Creator and of yourself, of your being and energy, healing and recharging all are occurring when you are living for the moment.

Examples of that are sweat lodges, pipe ceremonies, singing, praying, dancing, tai chi, going to church, meditation and yoga - anything which is spiritual and physical in combination creates living for the moment and then you feel much better about yourself, and happier because you have God in your life. And all of your parts are being taken care of.

So this is why living for the moment is quite important, because you make the right decisions, you let synchronicity flow freely and you are being used as a tool from the Creator much easier. You are less stressed, and you are more aware of life and the importance of life and its beauty. You are more aware of yourself, when you live for the moment, and you are happier. You look within yourself to find happiness, instead of looking outside, and this is what living for the moment creates.

Why People Do Not Change

The reason why people do not find or attain their goals, or look for their goals or achieve their goals, is because of the lack of understanding the process of this occurring, and also the unknown and uncharted territory of this journey.

They are afraid of the unknown and they are afraid of change. Even though they have a miserable life, they are afraid of change.

There are a few reasons why they are afraid of change. One is that they do not accept all aspects of themselves, and that is why they are afraid. They are not comfortable with every aspect of themselves. They push and deny the dark sides of themselves. The things that they think, not be in the norms of the positive society and so they push these down. Maybe they are unhappy, or do not want people to know about this part of them.

This also creates this lack of accepting all of you, for who you are and what you are - just trying to get reassurance from others about the things that you do that are good, and always wanting approval for the good things that you do, but always hiding the bad things that you do.

This is contradicting, so you never think that you are worthy of change or good things, or that you should work on change, because if you do change, then what happens next, is that you have to be responsible for that change. To maintain that change you have to be responsible for your feelings and the situation that comes with it - which is your purpose in life or a better, happier life. These responsibilities take work, devotion, dedication and sacrifice.

So these are the main reasons why somebody does not change or does not know why they do not change.

It is because subconsciously they know – maybe they are not aware of it upfront in their awareness, but somewhere back in their brain it is... well... I have to be kind and polite and respectful and be responsible for my own feelings, and my own thinking, and walk and grow up and with this purpose, that I find with myself, I have to have devotion, dedication and sacrifice, I have to work at it, I have to work for it, I am a tool now so that takes a lot of responsibility. If you hurt somebody's feelings you have to apologize, you have to be the first one to say "I am sorry", you have to swallow your pride, you have to have humbleness and humility, you might have to get up and exercise and eat better, and be more disciplined and change your way of life.

So it is a lot of work and some people are lazy - they do not want to do that.

So they say: "I am afraid of change", "I am afraid to change". But in reality they are not afraid. They think they are afraid, of change but what they are really afraid of is the responsibility, and the work that comes with change. The reason why they do not feel worthy of it, is that they do not accept the dark side of themselves, and say yes this is a part of me, and I am okay with that. Because socially it is not acceptable, they hide it. They put it away. Some people eat chocolate, some people have sexual fantasies, some people have addictions or something that they do not want other people to know that they do. Like smoke cigarettes, watch pornography on the computer, maybe cheating at poker or on paying taxes, or taking bribes or giving bribes to do something, or gambling, and nobody knows but them. So these are the things that they do not want other people to know.

So they do not accept that part of themselves. They hate it when they do that part, or they do not like that part of themselves, but it is a part of them so they need to accept it. Then they feel worthy, and that they are somebody special. Then they are worthy of, change and then they will try harder to change.

The Path of the Buffalo

A Perfect Life Circle

In order for an individual to have a healthy lifestyle, we first have to see a healthy human being and the process that this human being goes through – the patterns he goes through in his life circle.

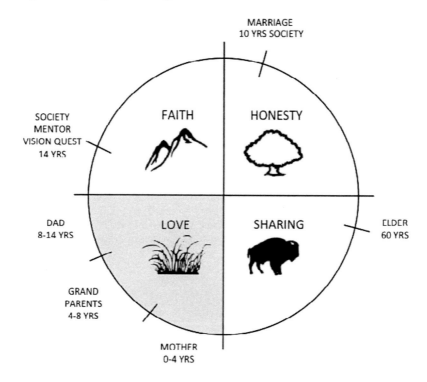

Childhood - Love

Mom

So you are born to a mother and a father, to a family, to a people and those first four years of your existence are basically with your mother. The father is there, and the rest of the family is there but the mother is the main constant caregiver in the first four years (whether it is your mother, father or grandparents, who is or are raising you).

An ideal mother in a perfect life circle is a mother, who is constantly there with the baby all the time. Mothers used to put the baby on their back when they worked, when they cleaned or tanned hide. The baby was always on their back wrapped in a blanket or in a cradle board. This way the baby was always near the mother, and she constantly had the baby with her.

In the first four years of life, you are developing the parts of your brain that will determine your being, when you grow up. All the love connections are being developed through eye contact, physical contact, gestures, expressions, love, hugging, protection, comfort and verbal phrases like "you are so cute" and "I love you". It is very important that the main caregiver does not express stress or anxiety, because these emotions also go to the child, reducing or stopping the healthy development of certain parts in of the brain. It can better connect to these love chemicals inside of you if the mother is not stressed.

These are the things that a child needs in its first stages of development, to develop proper brain function and is then less likely to need outside influences, to make them happy when they grow up.

The mother, of course, will set boundaries and not always give in to the child. As the child gets older, the child learns that there are boundaries, that the child should not cross, and he or she learns to behave properly from the mother.

The child learns in a proper way not to touch fire, a knife or something else that could hurt him. They do not always get candy, pop or whatever.

In the first four years of the child's upbringing, the mother should be giving the child constant care, constant reassurance, and should always be there to make the child feel secure, but at the same time she should not be overly protect of the child, and allow it to explore a bit. In that way the child learns to explore and trust itself, and do things on its own. This will be much needed, when the child is in his teens and as an adult, so that he can go out and achieve, seek and find things out and learn about life.

The mother is praying, and the child learns to pray sitting by the mother, father and grandfather. The mother sings for the child. She sings lullabies to rock him to sleep, sings a song when he is hurt, when he is sad or she sings songs of happiness, so that the child grows up with these songs, learning the songs from his mother. This enables the child to be able to sing to his own children later on, as well as sing for himself.

Singing is something that is lacking in the world today. When people do not sing, they block the connection to their spirit, to their soul, to their heart, to their mind, to the center of the earth and out into the universe. When people do not sing, they are blocked, so they do not get the messages they need to. The child is learning to sing, and they run around singing and they grow up singing, the adults are singing, the elders are singing. It is a part of life.

This is what a mother should be doing for a child. It is your mother creating the foundation, which establishes you as a healthy human being.

Umbilical Cord

All tribes had this philosophy of saving the umbilical cord and that was their connection to their mother, to their people and the connection to themselves. Every tribe had this belief system of the umbilical cord.

In the beginning you have your umbilical cord and in the Blackfoot way - the dried umbilical cord is put into a beaded pouch – usually of leather

– and is sewn shut and it is put on the baby's clothes… in front for the male and in the back for the female… the girl's pouch is a lizard and for the boy it is a snake. These two animals never get sick in life and that is why they use these.

Other native groups use different things like turtles and other animals, depending on their environment and their belief system. But everybody in the native world - at one time - saved the umbilical cord, and that was their connection to their family, to their loved ones, and to their mother.

Lack of Affection from Your Mom

If you do not get the proper affection from your mother or feel unwanted by your mom in some way or you feel rejected, it affects your belief that you are loved. Then there is a part of your brain that responds to that reaction. You do not get close to people, or allow people to get close to you because you are scared to be rejected again. If you feel they are rejecting you, not accepting or approaching you, then you sabotage the situation, or you make an excuse why it should not be this way, or with this person or whatever, so you run away from your emotions. It affects your ability to accept yourself, because your mother did not accept you in the way you feel she should have.

Grandparents

When the child is four years he is able to speak, to go to the bathroom, to express himself, to ask questions, to listen, to comprehend, and to understand. So at four a child is very encouraged to spend a lot of time with his grandparents.

The grandparents' job was to educate the child on life in an environment of living for the moment. Parents were busy trying to get food and keep the house in order, they had goals, they had dreams and they had cares.

But the grandparents had finished all of that, so they had time for the child, time for their questions, time for their dreams, time to explain things properly and this was about their relatives, who their relatives were, their original history, creation stories, constellations, stars, animal stories, plant stories, what was edible, what was not edible, animal behavior, what was dangerous, what was not dangerous, how to read nature, how to behave properly, the proper mannerism, to share, to understand that you belong to this collective group, which was the family, which was the tribe, which was the nation. You were the son or the daughter of this nation.

Pride was installed in the child, humbleness, humility, caring, loving, sharing all the positive attributes and this created roots within this individual. And of course the constant love from the grandparents as well.

The grandparents taught with love, caring and understanding and were the first ones to help the child understand what he or she was going through. The grandparents were able to give them advice because they were still learning to dream and imagine, and this was cared for and allowed to grow.

So imaginary friends and things to this nature were talked about and explained, and they understood this other world – the spirit world – where there were little people and the other spirit helpers, that come along and helped the people. These things were also taught to the child. They were exposed to how animals helped us.

Question: How do Animals and/or Spirits Help Us?

An introduction to nature and how to respect her and her being our mother was taught. Stories about Napi – our creation stories and all the mistakes Napi made and what he did wrong, which was quite funny listening to as a child. It taught us how to behave and how not to behave, through Napi's mistakes. It was our grandparent's job to tell us these stories about Napi – how he went through situations, and what to do and what not to do.

Then there were teaching on how the stars became like The Seven Brothers, and the story about the seven brothers and how that inspired us to dream, and to seek our own visions and goals in life. Also to call upon the seven brothers for help because we knew what they were, and what they stood for.

These were the things that we were taught by our grandparents as well as respect, especially respect around the spiritual people and the ceremonies themselves. Some of us were very fortunate to sit in the ceremony, when it was being done. We sat there with our grandparents, and learned as a young child, what was happening, and why it was happening. Usually these grandchildren are going to take their grandparents roles when they grow up, and continue the life of the medicine bundles[1] and caring for these bundles and sweat lodges.

Some of the grandchildren carried these traits of interest in our culture, and those were the ones who were encouraged to go to the ceremonies with their grandparents, and to sit and watch and learn and listen. These were the important moments; to be with your grandparents to learn how life works, and how nature works. The grandparents give their grandchildren an awareness and the attention that they did not give to their own children. They were busy working, and they did not give their children the time that they should have. So when they become grandparents, they spend that lost time with their grandchildren, and really teach them about these things that are so vital in a human being's life – to comprehend life, and to live life in a healthy way. It was done with such love and caring from the grandparents.

For this reason the grandparents were so important in a child's development. And of course the love and attention and the understanding, made the child feel human, because sometimes the child does not feel human: The child often feels that he in the way, the child gets pushed out of the way, told to be quiet and not to make noise. But when you are with yourgrandparents you are the center of attraction.

---

1 Medicine bundles are a significant part of Blackfoot culture and spirituality, preserving the songs and dances associated with ancient rituals.

Dad

In the first phase, the children are developing their heart, in the next phase, which is the teenage time, the mind is being developed.

The first phase went on until they were eight. They learned how to play with bow and arrows, and for the girls it was dolls and then they reached eight years old, and then they were being able to copy, admire and look up to people.

The first hero they had as a child was their father figure. The boys wanted to be like their dad. The girls started wanting to marry someone like their dad. They copied their dad's traits and abilities and tried to impress their fathers, getting their acknowledgement this way.

The father wanted to teach his sons and daughters about life, hunting, and what to find in the best marriage, the best way to be – by example. Whether they were warriors or shamans or whatever. This inspired the child and of course the affection and wanting to be accepted, was all taken care of.

With the dad the boy learned to wrestle. He was taught how to be a man by example, and his place in the community by how his dad presented himself. He gave the boy pride and the girl as well. His father's achievements inspired the boy to want to achieve like his father. They admired their father. They wanted to be like their father. The father taught them how to hunt, and how to use the weapons properly. He told the girl what to look for in a man, the good qualities of a husband, things the girl should watch out for.

These were the things and the responsibilities of the father taught to the child by example, how to lead a good life and bring them through a good life. Be the protector and provider, and they were teaching these boys and these girls how to manage the food, how to prepare it, how to store it, how to save it. The importance and the value of food, hunting and plants and all these things, were so important for the child to respect and to understand, and to learn, in order to survive in this harsh climate that they had to live in.

These were the things, they were taught by their father on respecting nature, respecting spirits, respecting animals and hunting laws, teachings and different things, that will make that child confident to hunt and to live, and know where to move to next, and how to find animal tracks etc.

So this child was learning these vital steps in transition, leaving the mother and coming closer to the father and slowly leaving the nest, which was the second phase of being a teenager. During this phase with your father, you slowly start transitioning away from mother and grandfather, being a little more strong and tough with father, and getting ready to be away from the family with friends, with society, spreading your wings and trying them out.

Dad Not There

You lack reassurance and self-esteem about yourself in certain ways. There was nobody there to say I love you, and I am proud of you, you did a good job, so you can become a perfectionist, and whether he was in your life, or never said it, or he was not in your life at all, you still need to hear it from your father's side. There is no way of getting around it. You need to adopt a father figure, to fill in that place of your father. And if your father was negative, and if it is hard to change or to get healing, between you and your father, it will take a long time. In the meantime you still need that change, so you adopt a father figure that will say "I love you" and "I am proud of you", and give you the positive things you need.

You can heal that part of you, and develop that part of you, that needs to be developed, so you can have a more positive outlook on life and yourself. You will achieve goals, and you will be satisfied with what you do, because if it is okay for them, then it is okay for you. This is the reason, why it is so important, to have a healthy father.

If you did not have a healthy father, then this is why it is so important to adopt a father. Because you are not going to change that part of you, by reading books and doing self-help. It only comes from the father part of your life. Once that is established, then healing and change occurs. You then believe in yourself a lot more or the way you do things changes and you find satisfaction and contentment, in what you are doing, instead of finding faults all the time.

Faith - Teenage Time

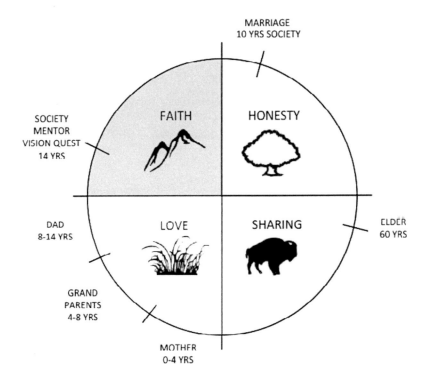

Then the child changed and went through a phase called puberty. The body started to change, hormones started to change. Attitude and outlook of life started to change in that individual. Now instead of just existing and doing what they wanted to do as a child, they started to see how other people viewed them. They started to have a sense of belonging to a group of their age. They wanted to have friends and the friends became important to them. They became teenagers.

You are looking at society. So there in your society you learn loyalty, friendship, discipline, honor, respect, challenge, brotherhood and then of course social skills, teasing, being teased, teasing back. Then you are busy—you belong to something.

I think that belonging is the biggest thing for teenagers. They are lonely and because you are an adult and you are losing all those things, mom, grandparents and dad, but in your mind you are still a teenager, you are not mature because you are a teenager and you still lack belonging to a group. That is why a lot of people are not social, or they do not know how to be social. They want to be. A lot of 20-30-year-olds are single, they do not belong to anything, but they want to belong to something. That should already have been taken care of when they were 14. They are 30, 40 or 50 and are still trying to belong. It is really important to fix that part. Then they can become a hermit, and not want anybody around.

Societies

A society should have a society name, a society song, and society colors. Then it should have rules, regulations, code of conduct, support, unity, goals and objectives. It must stand for something and be a protector in some respect and should set an example. A society should discipline its own members more than outside people.

In order for the teenager to go through this phase of change three things were implemented, so that child could have an easier transition into teenage life.

First is that they were put into age-grade-societies and these societies have been in place for centuries.

Then the young boys would join this new society at 14, be initiated into the society through ceremony, traditions and customs. These societies had rules, regulations and responsibilities to each other, and to the camp itself or the community. They had colors, and things they had to do. What was instilled in them was a unity – a brotherhood or a sisterhood. They had their society song, they had a society name, and they had rituals that they followed.

In the old days, there were different societies – for people of the same age – they called it: All Comrades' Society (Blackfoot name), and these societies would challenge each other to things like horse racing, foot races, gambling, war stories, and hunting. The different things they would challenge each other to, created entertainment for the rest of the camp.

Of course they would try to outdo each other, tease each other, and make fun of each other. That created within the society a discipline. And the societies disciplined each other.

So if one teenager,– for example, – was not listening to his parents the other members would come and say to that individual: "you are not listening to your parents, and if the other societies hear about this, we will all be teased because we do not listen to our parents". We do not want to be labeled like that. So you have to change. Otherwise we will kick you out, or whatever the consequences were.

From 14 to 19 your friends are your life. You do not want to be kicked out, so you change your attitude. This helps the parents in disciplining that teenager, because the societies took care of each other.

Mentor

The individual was also given or chose a mentor, somebody they looked up to, wanted to be like, admired or in who's footsteps they wanted to follow. The mentor could be someone who was in a profession that the child is interested in. A good mentor could be, for example, a great warrior, medicine man, mechanic, race car driver, sportsman - maybe a professional athlete, professor, veterinarian, doctor, craftsman or he or she could be a great winemaker.

It has to be somebody with a lot of achievements, who is really good at what they do. Whatever that mentor says, the teenager is going to take it to heart, and really think about it. Perhaps he follows that advice, or the examples he was shown. He will try to impress his teacher and himself, by changing something about himself. This is the purpose of a mentor. He is also there if you have problems, realizations, discoveries, desires or dreams. Your mentor is who you talk to. You ask him questions about life. It is somebody who is special in the eyes of the teenager, and therefore the teenager will listen to what he has to say.

Your mentor could be an uncle or another man in the camp. This was the person you went to when you had questions about life, questions about yourself, and questions about problems that you were going through. You were seeking advice and guidance from this individual. The mentor was not your parent, it was another person. It created an atmosphere of no. judgment. If you had a problem with girls or drugs or whatever, that person did not scold you or condemn you or give you a lecture about what you should or should not do. Instead they gave you choices to follow, and it was up to you to make your decision.

They gave you a couple of roads and examples of these roads: "if you follow this road this is what is going to happen, if you follow that road that is what is going to happen". So you had a choice from their own experiences of what to do, or what not to do. So you had the knowledge or an idea of what could happen, if you did this or did that.

Most times teenagers do not go to their parents with their problems – they go to somebody else. This is a very natural thing to do, and this is what the mentor is for.

A mentor should lead by example. He should be open, honest, supportive, understanding, a good listener, give advice and be patient. A mentor should have all these qualities.

A mentor should be someone to copy, ask questions of, and discuss problems with. You have someone to turn to when things are hard, someone to listen to you. Then of course there is the vision quest. You find yourself, your purpose in life, your connection to the universe and nature. You die and are reborn.

The rest of your teenage life is society, and living your purpose in life under an apprenticeship. Everything after that is a reflection of what happened in your childhood and teenage life.

Vision Quest

The other thing the parents or grandparents did for that individual at the same time, was to put him or her on a vision quest. That individual was given a pipe and was put on a hill or a mountain with a buffalo robe and a buffalo skull - some place sacred where the spirits would gather. That individual would sit there for four days and four nights without food or water trying to find themselves. Trying to find out what their purpose in life was. Why they were put here on earth. And they did that at a young age, because they were naive and did not have the scars, that life gives us.

In order to find yourself, you have to peel away all the layers and scars and walls you have created for yourself, because of negative experiences. In order to find your true self, and to find out what your purpose was, because your soul has the answer to your quest. Age 14 is a perfect time for an individual to find himself because he did not have to pull away so many layers.

He had a dream, or a vision of what he should be doing. He came down, and the medicine man would interpret, what it was that he was supposed to do. Then he went under an apprenticeship for the rest of his teenage life in conjunction with his mentor and society.

In the second Diagram of the Wheel, love is developed. Love for yourself and love for others. In the second state, which I have just been talking about, faith is created: faith in yourself, faith in others and faith in the Creator.

Adult - Honesty

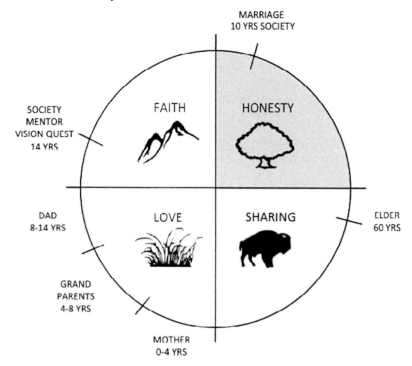

Then you became an adult, and that changed you as well. Honesty became important to the individual: trying to be an honest individual, trying to be honest with yourself, trying to be honest with others and expecting others, to be honest with you. Justice – all those things came into play.

Your purpose in life was being practiced at the same time. You got married and you started a family. Now understanding that you are not used to living with an individual like a partner maybe you had brothers and sisters, but that is a different relationship, compared to a husband or a wife. So you come together with another individual, and then you have to get used to living together. With different views perhaps, different outlooks, different behaviors and trying to combine them with yours, in order to become a strong couple.

At times you pretend to be interested in your partner's interests because you love them. So the man will pretend to be interested in the female's interests and vice versa. This is where the societies were very important.

Adult Society

Perhaps once a week you left your family unit and went to your society. There you vented about your relationship, you had others venting about theirs, and you saw a commonality there, which made you feel like you were not the only one, who was going through this deal, this situation or this problem. It made you feel a little bit more comfortable, that other people were having the same issues as you were.

Then you joke and laugh, and at the end you come to the conclusion as a society, that you cannot live without your partners.

Then you did things that the society was doing, and that you were all interested in, whether it was hunting, war stories, weapons – or for the women sewing or clothing or bead work or talking about kids or whatever. You were in your group again, talking about things that you were interested in, and they were as well. You were not pretending. After the meeting you felt fresh, revitalized and happy, which created within yourself a longing, to get back to your family. Then you guys got back together, and you became a better father, a better wife, a better mother, a better teenager, a better son or daughter, because you had a break from the family, and you were with like-minded people the same age as you, that understood the same things and felt the same things or similar things.

You conduct your life and carry on this way for ten years. After or during those ten years there comes another change which happens naturally. You start disassociating yourself with your childhood friends or society members.

Who becomes your best friend? Who becomes closer to you? Who are you finally sharing your secrets with? It is your partner. And they become your best friends because now you are used to each other. You had that ability to connect properly. You know each other's habits. You are used to each other by now. And your relationship is more solid and your love for each other is stronger. You know that this is your partner for life.

Then you join society together as a couple. And this is usually a sacred society where you by that time have acquired wealth, horses and gifts along your way.

You and your wife join this society, and you give away horses and blankets and goods for a sacred bundle, which is a sacred container with sacred items inside. This is what you use to have a good life and a good family. These bundles are thousands and thousands of years old and they are transferred down from generation to generation, with the law of that society and that bundle comes with it from the spirits. So you have to live a certain way and a certain lifestyle, to take proper care of these sacred objects. There are teachings you must follow. Women have their teachings and so has the husband as well as the children. There are certain things that you cannot do in the house anymore and there are certain things that you cannot touch anymore. This is all explained to the new members when they receive the transferring to this society.

So you get very connected to the bundle, and after four years or whenever, the society transfers the bundles to a new group of people. It is a lonely feeling: It is like you are giving up your child. Sometimes these couples will acquire another kind of bundle, and start living that life again, and they continue this lifestyle until they are around 60.

This system goes on until you are 60 for some individuals. After this you have acquired the knowledge and the understanding that bundles have to keep transferring from individual to individual throughout the tribe. The tribe owns the bundle, you don't own it.

You take these gifts and you go to the old members and you ask for their bundle. It is usually a sacred bundle. And your wife is very instrumental in this, and she is your helper. Then the transfer occurs from one society to the other, and then the bundle is transferred to you with all the education and meanings behind the bundle.

Now this bundle is a baby and it becomes your wife's responsibility to take care of this bundle. She carries the bundle. You as a man purchase the bundle. You come home with the bundle and you go to your society meetings and learn, and you have sweat lodges for the bundle.

People come to you throughout the year asking for help. You collect all these requests and the next year when you open the bundle, then the people who came to ask you for help throughout the year, have a chance to dance with these bundles to get better, and to fulfill their commitment, when they ask the bundle for help. This is the system. There are sweats and a lot of complex ceremonies that go with this system.

After the four years you transfer the bundle to a new society, which is like losing a child. You have become close to this bundle for four years. You feel for this bundle. It is your baby and then now you have to give it up. Of course that makes you lonely and sad, that you have to give this bundle up. Some individuals go and they get another bundle, whether they re-join that society or they take on a bundle from another society. Then they continue that life again. Now they have a new baby, and a new set of rules and they continue this life.

Elder - Sharing

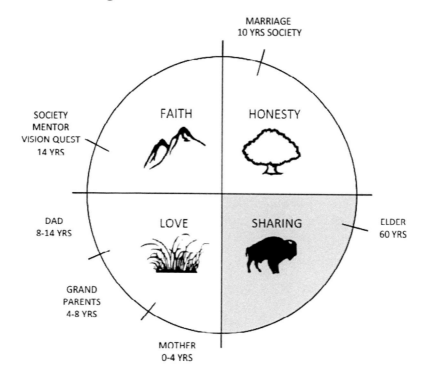

And so after this understanding and knowledge, and you become wiser. Your life changes again. Now you become an elder, a grandparent. Your attitude changes to sharing. Sharing your experience, your knowledge of life is when work really happens.

The child takes care of himself and only thinks about himself. The teenager is the same way – takes care of himself and only thinks about himself. The parent takes care of himself and the child. But the elder takes care of all three.

The grandfather gets up early, eager to teach his four year old grandchild something. Then perhaps the Grandfather is a mentor to one teenager, and perhaps he has to put another teenager on a vision quest. Then he has to go pick up his wife, and they go and do a ceremony in a society that they both belonged to, when they were younger.

The woman is educating the younger female on how to take care of the bundle properly, and the man is running the sweat lodge, for the males in that society. That is why elders are very much respected in our culture because they are the keepers of the knowledge for all the other phases of life. They have guidance and experience for each stage of life.

That continues till perhaps you are 80 and then you slow down. You start to forget things. You are not as strong as you used to be. You cannot sit up all night in a ceremony like you used to. You start forgetting songs – perhaps parts of the ceremony. So you retire and you let the younger elders run the ceremony. Perhaps you come to the first part of the ceremony because you enjoy it, but then you are older and you get tired, so you have to go home again. Then you complete your wheel.

Sometimes you start your wheel again. You are old enough. You become a child. You have to wear a diaper again, you repeat yourself, you don't like to be in the dark, you need to be held, you like candy again. You start your wheel again.

Those individuals are very lucky. They completed their wheel. They do not have to come back and do it again, so we are taught not to feel sorry for them, but to admire them. They made their journey in life complete holistically, and they started again. They will come back as spirit helpers. Other people do not complete their wheel, they have to come back and try it again.

Now what I explained to you, was a perfect lifestyle of an individual. If you lived this perfect life, your wheel will be centered, but of course today being the way it is we do not have this system in place. Many factors are not there to assure that an individual grows up healthy. You compare your life to this perfect life. You overlap it and then you can see where or what you did not receive properly.

Problems Rooted in Childhood

It could be in the early stage from zero to four, that you did not get the proper love or attention from your parent caregiver, or perhaps you did not get the proper teachings or educations from your grandparents or your first hero – your dad – was not a very good person to copy or follow, or have the proper things. A lot of factors come into play. Maybe early death of an individual like a grandparent or a parent, will stunt your growth. Then perhaps as a teenager, you did not have a society to belong to. Perhaps you did not have a mentor to go see with your problems. Perhaps you never went on a vision quest. So your heart has not developed properly, or your mind.

You become an adult, and you have no society to go to, when you and your wife are having difficulties getting used to each other. You are with them constantly. You get tired and separation occurs. Your parents try to discipline the teenagers. There is conflict. Then perhaps as an elder, you do not feel efficient enough, or that you have enough knowledge and self-esteem, to help the younger generations, because of the lack of education along the road that you lived.

So these are the problems we have today. The solution is to take it into your understanding of yourself that you need to put these things in order.

Perhaps you need to enable healing between your mother and yourself – by talking and understanding. Perhaps you need to reconnect with your grandparents, reconnect with your father, and of course every story is different. Maybe the parents do not want to heal this relationship, or maybe they are not healthy enough to do it or they are gone from this world. In those cases what you need to do, is to adopt healthy individuals – healthy parents, healthy and knowledgeable grandparents, or perhaps you need to join a society, or get a mentor. Perhaps you need to go on a vision quest in order to fill in these gaps.

Everything regarding your personal growth, understanding and healing starts from your childhood and teenage life. Everything after that - the adult and the old age part – is a reflection of what happened in the first two parts of your life. So in order to change when you are 35 or 42 – you have to realize that your problems started when you were younger. You cannot change them with what is in front of you now. You have to go back and heal those things or fix those things. Once those things from your past are in place or healed properly, then you will mature where you are at today.

The adult life is a reflection of what you experienced, when you were young. If when you were young you saw your mom and dad fighting a lot, chances are that when you grow up, you will also fight and argue a lot with your partner.

You will copy your parent's good qualities and bad qualities. You will copy your grandparent's qualities as well. This is a natural state for any human being. We learn by copying.

So when we are of age to have children, it is already programmed in us

– through copying – how to be a parent. From our experience with our grandparents, we learn how to be a grandparent to our grandchildren. If our grandparents have negative behaviors, then it only makes sense to copy a healthy elder to reprogram ourselves. Then we will become a healthier parent or grandparent and a healthier partner to our spouse. This is how we fix this particular medicine wheel.

Adopting

Of course everybody does not grow up with the perfect lifestyle. We have a lot of problems with our upbringing, whether it was a lack of affection from our mother or we did not have the proper love, the proper education and the affection that we needed for our brain to develop properly. The receptors in our brain may not have connected properly, due to the lack of constant intimate care.

Maybe we have problems with our grandparents. Perhaps they are not there to show us these things, or maybe they are there, but they do not show us the traditions, the culture or the customs. So we lack in those two areas. Then there is the father. Maybe we were scared of him, he got mad or whatever the father was doing.

They were not always positive role models. There was arguing and fighting that you witnessed as a child.

Low self-esteem due to not fitting in, lack of societies, lack of proper attention and teachings create a very lonely child. Growing up we tend to

The Path of the Buffalo

make walls that shield these scars. What we need to do, is to reopen the scars and feel safe to reopen them. We are around a person or people that make us feel safe, to open up our feelings and express them properly and in a healthy way. But it is not just one person who does this. You need people that model certain characteristics of a mother, grandparents and the different levels of love, you receive from a parent and a grandparent. Then there is also an adopted father to get positive things from. That will help change the heart.

Then you think about faith in yourself, faith in others and trust and all these types of things. It is good to be in a society, have a mentor and also fix all the things you need to fix. Then perhaps going on a vision quest when you are ready will help.

All these things will help an individual correct themselves today. Whether they are 25, 30 or 40 they can still turn around and fix things that they have gone through. Comparing their life and their family's story to the positive life style, and then seeing what they are missing, and then filling those in or fixing them or healing them. There are many ways to look at a situation, and change it. They can see the difference afterwards with past behavior, in relationships and in the family and among friends.

Traumas

It takes a lot of changes and a lot of awareness about yourself, in order to change things that are harmful or not good for you into something positive. Sometimes the only way you will get those, is if you copy somebody – copy their behavior and hang around them and copy that. It is the only way. So if you adopt these parents and grandparents etc., you are setting yourself up for the initiation of copying these people and becoming like them. So choose good people and you will change to be like them.

There were many different situations when you grew up with parents and grandparents – parent caregivers. Sometimes you did not know how to handle the situation. Perhaps you grew up with one parent because the other parent died, or you grew up with a single parent, and you do not know the other parent. There are many different situations, where there is trauma and closing down because of a situation and you block things to protect yourself. So you close up. At times there is no one there to tell us how to handle the situation. We were not prepared.

There is blame, and there is guilt. There are many things that go through an individual's mind towards their father or mother or grandparents. It is a touchy subject. First of all you have to understand, that you cannot change anybody else's way of thinking. You can only change your thinking and hope – by example – you change another person's thinking – by showing the example first. If you want to have somebody who is trustworthy, you have to make people feel trustworthy. Then you will get it in return.

There are a lot of positive people out there, who would be good adopted parents or grandparents – people that would be good role models to copy in order to change the way you are. The hard thing is to find them, or to ask them, or to get to know them.

That is when you make an offering to the Creator - something valuable. Then you wait for four days to get a direction, which you then follow. Things will come up, and you will deal with them as they show up.

Many people get stuck in those areas because they do not properly follow the protocol. The protocol is to have faith in what you are asking for, and believing that it will happen. A lot of people give up, or have different expectations. Sometimes they do not see the answer.

We all have to go through this learning process to come to an understanding at some point down the road as to how it works properly. What we have to do is heal ourselves today – the blockages in us. We are afraid to have a partner and a family. Yet we want these things even though we are afraid to have them. There are a lot of factors in that, but you look back and you see the way your parents were to you. If you did not feel wanted, chances are that it is pretty hard for you to want a baby. These are the things that get stuck in us because of how we grew up. So coming to deal with a situation, we want something and we do not want it.

But people have to make a choice. They have to make a decision of what they want to do in their life. If they want to change their marriage status and become healthier, then they should fix their parents and their relationship with their parents, whether they are alive or dead. Talk to them at the grave or talk to them alive. Change your relationship through them – forgive and understand. Then you stop that pattern from being copied by your kids. They will copy something else.

The Path of the Buffalo

We change in order to feel better about ourselves, and to have a different heart towards the people that are closest to us. We also want to open our hearts towards ourselves in order to love ourselves and be happy with ourselves.

Now we go to the Second Diagram:
The Wheel has Grass, Rocks, Trees and Buffalo

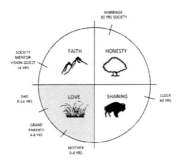

Grass

If you go to the first part of the wheel the representation is grass. As a child you have to understand that there is grass that will nourish you, grass to make incense with and grass for smudge. We call it sweet grass. These are the positive grasses that will heal you, nourish you or teach you. Then there are also the poisonous grasses that you stay away from, because they could harm you, make you very ill or perhaps you could even die from digesting them. There are also the grasses that irritate your skin. These are the grasses that you have to be aware of and know to stay away from.

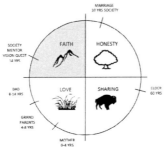

Rocks

Then we go to the teenage part. That is the rocks. We use rocks for many things such as to make pipe stones, and in the sweat lodge. Lava rocks are used to heal people and to doctor people. We also use rocks to pray with. Certain rocks are holy rocks like a buffalo stone, and certain rocks that you find are sacred. We get the healing from these rocks.

Then there are rocks that can harm you like obsidian – arrow heads, - sand stone rocks which can explode in the sweat lodge, or rocks which they fashion into weapons. So you have to understand and respect the two kinds of rocks.

Trees

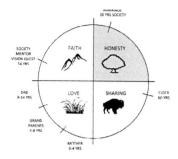

When you go to the tree and the adult section you experience the honesty of a tree.

There are trees that we use for spiritual things like center poles or smudging. Some trees have fruit on them which we eat and nourish ourselves with. Some trees are used to build homes with. Some are used for firewood to stay warm or to cook with.

Some trees are medicine trees, so we use the bark to doctor ourselves and mix with tobacco and pray with. We make bows with other trees. Then there are other trees, which are harmful to you. The trees are poisonous. You have to understand the different trees and respect them as well.

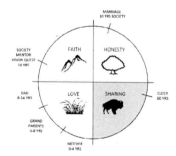

Animals

When we go to the elder's part of the wheel, the representation is an animal. There are animals out there, that will give you gifts and dreams, and provide food for you, as well as heat, warmth, protection or transportation, but then there are also the other animals that could harm you. They could bite you or poison you or try to eat you. They are not there as your friends, they are trying to dispose of you in some way. They are angry animals. You have to know the difference between the animals too and respect them. Not all animals are spirit animals that are there to help you.

Negative and Positive Parts of Ourselves

Now you understand the two kinds – the ones that could help you and the ones that could hurt you.

Then we start to look at ourselves and there are two parts of us. There is the positive part that tries to do good things, but then there is also the dark side of us that we try to hide from people, we put it in the closet and do not want people to know about it. That is a part of us too and sometimes we are ashamed of it, sometimes we get addicted to it, but that is a part of us.

Some people try to suppress this part, and then it blows up. When you want to change and evolve into a better human being, many people make the mistake of just going there with their positive side, and still not accepting the negative or the dark side of themselves, and saying yes this is a part of me.

They cannot fully change. They cannot fully go to the next step or level, because they are leaving a part of themselves behind. When you move to another section, you have to take all of you to the next section.

Becoming friends with the negative side of you, and accepting that, this is who you are enables you to control that side and suppress it when you need to.

That is called unconditional love of yourself, and once you have unconditional love of yourself, then you understand why your partner or your children love you unconditionally. We are our own worst critics and we do not see what other people see in us.

We always condemn ourselves and beat ourselves up for making mistakes. We look in the mirror and we wish we looked different. We want to look different.

But then our partners look at us, and they love us for who we are, and so do our children. They accept the good part of us, and the negative part of us as a whole being, and they love us like that, and we do the same for them, but we cannot do it for ourselves. Therefore accepting the negative part of, yourself is a step forward to accepting yourself unconditionally.

The Path of the Buffalo

When you go on the mountain you go up there with expectations of getting your purpose in life but if you have not by that time accepted the negative side of, yourself and made it your friend, then all you will be doing is realizing yourself and seeing yourself. All you will get up there is a realization of yourself, a realization of the world, the plants and everything around you but you will not get your life purpose.

When you accept the negative side of, yourself and you are okay with it, before you go up the mountain, then your purpose can be revealed to you, because not only do you accept the negative side of yourself, which makes you able to change into a healthier person, you also have fixed your insecurities with your parents, grandparents, mentors and society. Everything is in check and growing to a healthy stage, and everything seems to be going in a good way. Accepting the negative side of yourself you then are able to change and to see your purpose in life. Lacking some of these things will have great impact on you finding your purpose in life, or getting a dream to doctor people etc.

Examples of Second Diagram of the Medicine Wheel

Childhood

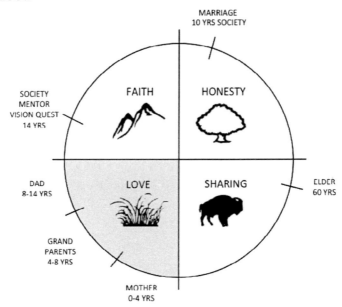

MARRIAGE
10 YRS SOCIETY

SOCIETY
MENTOR
VISION QUEST
14 YRS

FAITH

HONESTY

DAD
8-14 YRS

LOVE

SHARING

ELDER
60 YRS

GRAND
PARENTS
4-8 YRS

MOTHER
0-4 YRS

Development of Love or Heart:

In the first section the first component consist of four years. From 0 to 4 years the child should be with the mom. She should be available and give constant care and attention to the child. This important time with the mother helps to create proper brain development for self-care. It also provides, love, acceptance, security and stability. This is what is created, by being with your mom for the first four years. Being around your mom through eye contact helps to create the proper brain function, the proper opiates and endorphins and stress relief.

Through hugging, constant attention, constant affection and constant love, the child learns to take care of himself, so that down the road they have the proper endorphins to deal with stress, loneliness, sadness without having to drink, take drugs or take a pill. Their body is creating all these things for itself so that they do not need outside influences to make them feel better due to proper development.

We are going through the perfect life…

Grandparents

The child is able to walk, comprehend, use the bathroom on their own and can communicate. The child lives for the moment and so do the grandparents. They communicate on the same level.

The child is taught about his roots, identity, clans, relatives, creation stories, songs, rituals. He is taught how we fit into the circle of life, our relatives: the animals and plants, how we fit in and are related to them, how to pray, how to communicate properly and how to behave properly. Our grandparents prepare us for the future by telling us what to look out for growing up. So they are telling you that in the future when you run into alcohol, drugs or women this is what you do and do not do. You are just a kid but you already have a pre-plan given to you for the future. The grandparents also teach the child how to make things. As children we help grandpa make a drum or skin a deer and help grandma bake bread and help in the garden, and then later on we know how to do these things.

The child goes hunting and gathering food with them learns to make medicines and accompanies them to ceremonies.

Dad

Dad is our first hero. Boys copy their father and daughters want a partner like their dad. We imitate our father and take on his belief system on life or parts of it. So if your dad complains about the government when you are growing up, then when you grow up, you will complain about the government. If your dad has an attitude towards certain kinds of people, then you will too. Once you meet those people you may change your attitude towards them.

We do copy some things from our dads and other things we change into our own philosophy, if we do not agree with them on that particular subject.

Example:
If your dad is a racist towards black people, and you grew up and were a racist as a little kid, then later on you meet a black person, and you become friends, then you change your attitude towards black people, then your mindset is different than your dad's. But on another note your dad is complaining about the government, and you continue to complain. So

we do copy some of their belief systems, and in others we make our own.

We get security and determination from our dad's actions. We want his approval and love. It is which are essential for the outcome of our actions in the future, and how we conduct ourselves.

So if we get approval from our dad and we receive love and he says: "You did a good job", "I love you son", "I am proud of you, son" then you will be proud of yourself and be content with whatever you do, whether you are working or building a deck at home.

You will be happy with your work, because your father is good with you. But if he never said "you did a good job" or "I am proud of you" then what will probably happen is that you will become a perfectionist and nothing will be good enough for you.

We learn to be proud of ourselves through our dad's achievements and actions, and we want to follow in his footsteps.

Example:
You are happy and it makes you proud because your dad was a chief. You feel good and important too. This makes you want to have a headdress down the road. It sets your goals higher when you see your dad achieve things.

From 8 to 14 is the time when it is important that you spend time with dad, and it is also the time you start school.

The elders will make all the children run to see who the fast ones are and they will leave the fast ones alone. The elders will work with the slow ones, until they are just as fast as the fast ones. If there is a child who just cannot run then the last resort of the elder is, that he is given the personal power of the elder. Now that child is faster than the rest. No one is left behind. This goes for other teachings from other elders in other situations.

The Path of the Buffalo

Faith

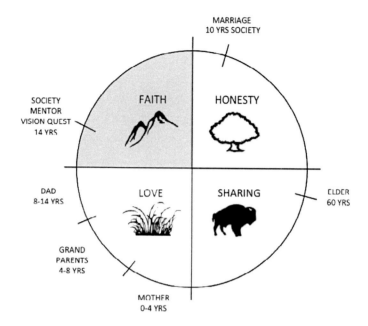

Now we go Into the Teenage Development.

At 14 you need a society:

So at 14 you are changing from being a child to being a youth. You are going through puberty. Your hormones are changing as are your body and your voice. You are slowly separating from your parents and grandparents and are starting to look outside the family borders. Now your attention goes towards friends and the opposite sex.

Society provides a sense of belonging: Same age, same gender, you have colors, rituals, society songs, rules and regulations and duties towards your community. You belong and have things to do.

The society also disciplines one another.

Example:
If one member does not listen to his parents the other members will confront him and tell him to change because the society does not want to be labeled as not listening to ones parents. He or she decides to change instead of being kicked out. From 14 to 19 your friends are your life.

There are older societies, which you challenge, for example horseracing, warrior stories, hand games and other contests. These activities create unity in the society and they encourage the members to develop skills. They also creates entertainment for the community.

Mentor

A mentor will mentor the teenager if he accepts, then the youth will seek advice from that person. If the youth was lazy, then the parents will ask the mentor to talk with them. He will tell the youth stories about his experiences, and how he tried hard and this will encourage the youth to try harder because he wants to be like his mentor.

So the mentor is there to encourage the child, listen to him when he has problems, talk to him about girls or guys or whatever. At the same time the mentor is an example. You see how the mentor gets things, how he looks upon life, how he expresses himself and does all these things. Those are lessons you want to take and utilize for yourself in your own personal endeavors in life. You see how the mentor looks look upon things. Then you copy those things so that you can do your work with a positive attitude and faith and asking Creator. All these things you copy from the mentor.

There is more about the mentor later, but that is a start.

The Vision Quest

At 14 the youth is ready to go on his own to a spiritual place to seek a vision, which will include his purpose in life and direction as to what he or she will become. He is sweated in the sweat lodge and given a pipe and he will fast for four days. When he comes down from the vision quest, the elders will interpret his dreams and experiences to determine what he will become. Afterwards he will go under an apprenticeship of someone, who is already doing this in order to learn from that person's example. It could be: healer, warrior, herbalist, leader, craftsman or a teacher. So you would go under one of these apprentices and learn from them.

Adult

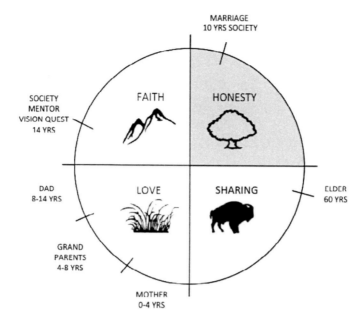

As an adult you start acquiring things and you get married. You are not used to living with someone, so you try to be interested in their interests. That is when your society is important. You go to your society to do things with them, and have a break from your marriage. When you are home you are re-energized and you are a better husband, a better father, a better wife, a better son or daughter.

After ten years your wife becomes your best friend, and your teenage friends are less important. Then you join a society together with your spouse, where all the other members are couples, and it is usually a spiritual society. Here you learn to take care of a bundle or a pipe. The wife smudges and takes care of the pipe or bundle as well. When you transfer the bundle or pipe it is a lonely time, so you take another bundle or pipe. This continues until 60 and you become an elder.

Elder

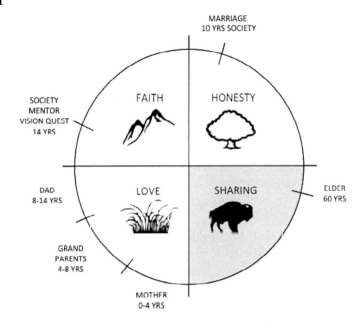

MARRIAGE
10 YRS SOCIETY

SOCIETY
MENTOR
VISION QUEST
14 YRS

FAITH

HONESTY

DAD
8-14 YRS

LOVE

SHARING

ELDER
60 YRS

GRAND
PARENTS
4-8 YRS

MOTHER
0-4 YRS

After 60 years of age you are an elder. Now you start to work. You have to teach the 4-year-old grandchildren and be a teacher as well. Then you are a mentor helping with sweats and society ceremonies. You take care of the adults, and you and your wife take care of sacred societies. She teaches the wife and he teaches the husband about sweats and the bundle. This work continues till you are 80, then you retire. At that time the younger elders take over your previous work. You come for a small part of the ceremony or pow wow, and go home early because you are tired. Sometimes you complete the circle and you start again. Then you become like a child; you like candy; you wear diapers; you need to be held; you repeat yourself and you forget. You should not feel sorry for these people, because they completed their wheel. They will come back as spirit helpers in the sweat lodge and heal people. If you do not complete your wheel, or left things out of your wheel then you will come back and try again.

The Path of the Buffalo

Self Evaluation

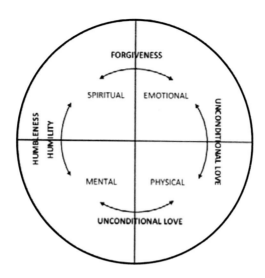

The 3rd. Diagram is the Self-Evaluation. Then how does the body function. Next is how to transfer energy by the bridges.

Five People Will Stop You from Changing

There is one thing you have to understand when you change. When you fix these things with your parents you completely change. Then you are not the same person that you were yesterday, so there is a shock that occurs with your family, your wife, your children and your friends. Now you are a different person because you have healed things. Sometimes others are not ready for such an abrupt change in you.

Therefore it is always important to make your partner aware of what you are trying to do, and what you would like to have happen after the change. Maybe it is a pleasant surprise, and other times it is not, because the wife or the husband are used to a certain way of living, and was comfortable with it and now it is different. Maybe you are surer of yourself. It may create insecurities for your partner. You might leave them because you are up, ready and willing to change things in your life, career and goals. There is always this fear that you might leave because of your new awareness. There has to be stability and reassurance to your partner when you initiate change.

Another thing is: that in order to change, there are five people you have to overcome. There are five people that might create obstacles for you to stop you from achieving your goals.

The first one is you yourself. The second one is your spouse, who does not want change. Then your children, your parents and your brothers and sisters. The last ones Is your closest friends. These will be the people who will try to stop you from changing, because they are used to you the way you are today.

Open Heart

The purpose of having an open heart is really quite simple: To be happier and have a happier life. Not a life of worrying, fear, doubt, wondering and asking "what am I doing here?" "Is there more to life than this?", I am lonely", "I want this" and "I think this will make me happy" and "I do not know what I want", "I do not know what I need". All those feelings are eliminated when you love yourself. Of course they linger, but you can overcome them. They do not consume you and run your life.

When you are happy and you have an open heart, you have the ability to want to explore, want to discover, you are curious, you can express your feelings, you are free, and you are not restricted from things that restricted you before. You are free to hug and receive hugs. You feel that joy, that happiness from it. You are happy, you give love, you look at things and life positively, you pray, and you have a sense of direction in a good way. This is why it is really important to have an open heart. It enables you to find your purpose in life, the job you want you are happy. You find a partner and you make each other happy, and you have a family if you want to. It is healthy and the right way to be. Then you have a healthy mind and a healthy heart. You are close to your soul, you are close to the creator, you are close to nature, you are close to people and you are close to yourself. This is why it is important to be happy. The way to get an open heart is: to forgive people and copy people. That is how you open your heart.

If you come from a place where people's hearts are closed it is difficult to find a way to open your heart. There is nobody there to copy from, but if you go to another country, where people have open hearts, and they are loving, affectionate and caring, you will have someone to copy. It will feel weird in the beginning, but eventually you will get used to it living with an open heart. Then you start living that way and it will become a part of you, and you can do it openly without fear, because people are showing you by example how to do it. You are learning by watching and mimicking or copying their gestures.

Perhaps the first time you hug somebody it feels strange and weird, but the more you hug people as you go along, the more comfortable you become with it. Then pretty soon it feels right to hug, and you feel good doing it. You cannot learn all this from reading a book. You need to be around people who express this feeling, and who have an open heart. There will be resistance at first. It will be hard to understand the feeling, it will be weird, but pretty soon you just slowly adjust to it. It will become part of you, and then it is good for you to do that.

People who have an open heart can express their feelings, they can express themselves, they can talk about themselves, they can show you the good part and the bad part of themselves, and you can see it in their interactions with other people: they cry and they laugh. You can see that they have an open heart. If a person is stone cold, not hugging anybody, not expressing his feelings, not talking about himself, not talking about anything, and when he is talking about people it is always negative, that person has a closed heart.

A person cannot say that he is a spiritual guide and teacher, if he talks negatively about people and has a closed heart. That is contradictory. You need an open heart, to have a proper connection to the creator. If you do not have an open heart it is hard to get dreams, it is hard to get answers, and it is hard to get a connection. That is why a lot of people have a hard time on vision quests, or looking for their purpose in life. Maybe the reason the tree ceremony does not work for them is because they do not have an open heart. You keep telling them, that they need to have an open heart. They do everything else except what they need to do, and everything except what is the key to open these things. This is what they have to realize and discover or be told. The questions and examples always go back to these same things: forgive and copy healthy people. There is no way around it. Every question goes right back to the same things, no matter what.

Over-Loving

If you were not around your parents growing up then you were very lonely which traumatized you. So when you have your children, then you keep them close. You love them, you do everything for them, and you do not let them go without. At every turn you are there to pick them up, to comfort them, to love them, to support them, to do things for them and to take care of them.

They grow up with a lot of love and affection, but they do not have the ability to do things for themselves, because you did not teach them how to do that. Maybe you never really said "no!" to what they wanted, so they are used to having anything they want without restrictions. They grow up expecting that from other people. Later they get very disappointed or upset from colleagues, or society because they were spoiled. They expect everything, and they do not know how to work for it. They just expect it. So over-loving your children could be a problem too, because these effects happen. There has to be a balance where there is both love, and affection as well as discipline where the parents are able to say "no" to the child.

Dad

Sometimes dads have a hard time expressing love in a healthy way, or expressing their pride in their children. They will say: try harder, you can do better, you can get a better grade. In most cases the dad cannot even reach those expectations, so what he is trying to say to the child is: "I want you to have a better life than me. I do not want you to be stuck doing what I am doing. I want you to be a doctor, a lawyer or a brain surgeon, so try harder. You can do better than a B+, you can get an A+."

So that is their way of encouraging their child. It is their way of saying: "I love you", "I am proud of you" and "try harder." Of course it is not understandable to the child. He feels the opposite. He feels that nothing he does is good enough for his dad.

What could happen if that is what you experienced, is that you become a perfectionist and nothing is good enough for you. Even though people comment on your good work and the quality of the work you do, you will always find faults with it. It will never match your expectations, because you do not have reasonable expectations. You are always striving to be better than what you are, because your dad was pushing you. Only the day when your dad says: "I am proud of you, you did a good job" only then you will stop being a perfectionist. Then you will accept your work, as good quality work and stop finding fault with it.

So we really need this healing and realization from our father and from our mother as well. This is another way of parents saying "I love you" to the child, without saying it directly.

And of course the child misinterprets this and thinks: my parents never really supported me or loved me. They always expected more than what I could do. Nothing was good enough for them. You get these resentful feelings and feelings of rejection. Then the outcome is that you will never do it, the work you were meant to do. You do not believe in yourself, or you lose faith in yourself, or you give up. The opposite could happen and you become a perfectionist.

These things can happen. So talking to your parents, having them express their love, gratitude and pride in you, will eliminate some of these walls that you created for yourself and change some of your negative belief systems. It will enhance your faith in yourself, the security within yourself, your ability to try things and your effort to accomplish things.

Supporting Dreams

Your parents and grandparents should be supporting you through love and encouraging you. It is healthy for a child to play out his fantasies whether it is by stomping around like a dinosaur or pretending to be a fairy godmother or a princess. Allowing the child to play out the fantasies without restrictions or being put down assists them in dreaming. Sometimes we buy them princess clothes or a dinosaur shirt, and we encourage them to act out and play out their fantasies and roles.

It gives them dreams and desires for the future. As they grow up they have an Idea of whether they want to become this or they are better at that. They may want to experiment or do try something different.

Because they had support and encouragement as children, they feel safe to try out that new experience, without allowing their fears to hold them back. They believe in themselves, so they go for that change or that goal or that experience later in life.

That is why it is so important as the child is growing up, that the parents and the grandparents really support them, and encourage them to fantasize, to play and to dream. That is where dreams come from, and how they develop and create, so that further down the road when you are older, you have these dreams and desires which are not impossible. They become possible.

Parents and grandparents have supported the child and encouraged them to be what they want to be, and that is what their dreams are. If they change their minds later it is their own responsibility to become aware of that and to make the change. All you can do is support them and their dreams, and what they would like to do. You have to support the child and their dreams as a parent and a grandparent.

Why Change Does Not Occur

The reason why people do not find, attain, look for or achieve their goals, is because of the lack of understanding the process of this occurring and the unknown, and uncharted territory of this journey. They are afraid of the unknown and they are afraid of change. Even though they have a miserable life, they are still afraid of change.

There are a few reasons why they are afraid of change. One thing is that they do not accept all of themselves and that is why they are afraid. They are not comfortable with every aspect of themselves. They push and deny the dark side of themselves, the things that they think of that are not in the norm of the positive society. So they push these feelings down. Maybe they are not happy, or do not want people to know about this part of themselves so they do it when people are not looking. They are not happy about that part of themselves, and so they do not accept all of themselves.

When you do not accept all of yourself you try to get reassurance from others about the things that you do well and you always want approval for the good things you do, but are always hiding the bad things, that you do.

This is contradictory so you never think that you are worthy of change or good things, or that you should work on change because if you do change then what happens next is that you have to be responsible for that change. To maintain that change, you have to be responsible for your feelings and the situation that comes with it, which is your purpose in life, or a better, happier life. That responsibility takes work, devotion, dedication and sacrifice.

So these are the main reasons why somebody does not want to change, or does not know why they do not change. Subconsciously they know. Maybe they are not aware of it up front in their awareness but somewhere in the back of their mind the person is thinking "I have to be kind, polite, and respectful and be responsible for my own feelings and my own thinking and walk and grow up and with this purpose, that I find for myself. I have to have devotion, dedication, sacrifice, I have to work at it and work for it. I am a tool now." That takes a lot of responsibility. If you hurt somebody's feelings you have apologize, you have to be the first one to say 'I am sorry'. You have to swallow your pride; you have to have humbleness and humility. You have to get up and exercise, eat better, and be more disciplined as well as change your way of life.

So it is a lot of work and some people are lazy: they do not want to do that. So they say: "I am afraid of change!" But in reality they are not afraid, they just think they are. What they are afraid of is the responsibility and the work that comes with change.

The reason why they do not feel worthy of, the change is because they do not accept the dark side of themselves, and are aware of it and accept it and say "yes this is a part of me, and I am okay with that" because socially that is not acceptable. So they hide it and put it away. Some people eat chocolate, some people have sexual fantasies, some people have addictions or something they do not want other people to know, that they do. Maybe they smoke cigarettes or watch pornography on the computer or whatever. It can be many different things. It could be cheating at poker or with on their taxes, taking or giving bribes to do something, maybe gambling and nobody knows but them. So these are the things that they do not want other people to know. They do not accept that part of themselves. They hate it when they reveal their dark side. They do not like that part, but it is a part of them, so they need to accept it. Then they feel worthy and that they are somebody special. They feel worthy to change, and then they will try harder to change.

Early Skills

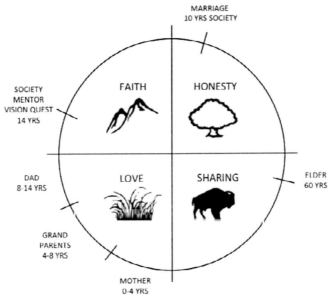

Love Mom

When we look at mom, there are a lot of factors that mom has to contribute to your security within yourself. Many of those memories are not the memories that you recall, they are the memories that your brain recalls or your body recalls.

You do not remember back to when you were one or two. You do not remember being rejected or being lonely or being left alone. You will remember that after the age of three or four. It is working on the implicit memory, the memory of your body and your brain. Those receptors in your brain are not getting the things they need if you are not getting your love and affection. Your interest, your drive and your motivation are not being fed. All these things are not being developed properly: Your self-esteem, your self-confidence and being accepted, being loved, being wanted and feeling it from the other person.

Of course everybody has different experiences with their parents depending on the parent with the child. Some parents really hugged their children and carried them around, some bossed them around while others were really strict, and showed no affection. Some children received a lot of affection. So you grow up with different characteristics, a different outlook on the world and different levels of going for it, of being assertive or having that courage or that belief in yourself to go do something like exploring or trying to get something. Some kids just sit back and do not go for it. They wonder how other kids can do it while they cannot. It is because their parents were raising them a certain way, and they grew up with these characteristics.

It is the other one who did not get them. They have to work to get them. Let us say that in the Indian world people really love their kids and they hug them. Then you look at European raised kids, or something like that, and you compare those kids. One of them will not have love and the other one will. So they will grow up differently and how they see themselves will be different too. An Indian on the reserve may not have much money but he has love. If he goes on the mountain and you get a kid from Europe and you put him on the mountain too, they are each going to have a different experience because of the way they were brought up, and the way they were taught to look at themselves. And that from a mother to child development and affection all that stuff all that was part of it too. You are looking at a lot of important situations that made that baby feel loved or not loved.

All babies act the same – no matter where you are in the world. They are in tune with their dark side which is why they are pure. You are sitting there watching two babies, and one will grab a toy and will just play with it, then the other one cries because he wants that toy, and the baby who does not have the toy will hit the other baby. That other baby will cry or hit back and if he is bigger then he will always get the toy. That it is already established. There is a pecking order between brothers and sisters. –You know that there is a pecking order between wolves. All over the world is the same human, natural way of being – the purest form of we are. When we are brought up we are made aware of those things. Some cultures teach you to deal with your feelings through stories and stuff while others do not really do that.

Napi[2]** went to the water and he saw these berries, so he dove in and he saw the berries in the water, but he could not get to the bottom, so he tied rocks on his hands and feet, and he jumped in the river and he sank to the bottom but on the bottom all he found was sand. There was nothing, so

---

[2] Napi is frequently portrayed as a trickster, a troublemaker, and a foolish being, but he is also responsible for shaping the world the Blackfoot live in, and would frequently help the people or teach them important knowledge.

he had to cut himself free from the rocks and get got out of the water. By that time he is choking and gasping for air, and he crawls up on the beach and he is coughing up water and then finally he lay on his back, and there above him are the berries. Then he gets so mad, and he took a stick and he starts hitting the tree. He was mad at it – because he almost drowned, – and then the berries fell. That is how they pick that certain kind of berries from that story.

So in our upbringing when we are little kids we hear that story, and we think: "boy that Napi is stupid". How come he did not know that the berries are above him, and not in the water? That was a reflection. Then we start to understand that he thought that the berries were there, but they were not really there. So when we grow up and look at situations we start to think is it there, or is it not really there? Does that person really love me, or is the love not really there? So you feel out your aunties and uncles and friends and boyfriends and girlfriends that way. You learn about it through Napi and the berries. And we still pick berries. It is always a reminder. And in other cultures there are other children stories that reflect the same thing, I am sure.

You get over it quickly as a child if you got rejected, but that memory stays in you. Maybe you were abandoned – your mom went to the store for a couple of hours and you were just crying, crying and crying. Finally when they came back you forget about it. You do not even remember. But that traumatized you and you are always crying when you see them leaving. They always come back, but babies do not know that. You go around the corner and they think you are gone. They cannot focus and visualize that you are around the corner, they just think you disappeared. It is not until they get a little older that they start looking around the corner. So when they see you putting on your jacket, they do not think that you are going to come back. They think that you are gone forever. Then later on, they start thinking, that you will come back, but not when you are really small. That is why you cannot have your mother always going away.

When your mother is around you she cannot be stressed out. If she is stressed out then you will always be stressed out as an adult. Stressed out about your relationship or job or whatever, because your parent was stressed. So to get unstressed you need to hang around people, who are not stressed out. Then you will learn not to become stressed out. So you have to adopt a mom who is not stressed.

That is one scenario. Another one is mom never hugs you, so you adopt a mom that hugs. And then you hug this mom all the time and then when you go see your own mom, you hug her and it is kind of strange, but it feels good, and then you guys make that a tradition. You brought it home. So that is a copying right there. Or saying 'I love you' or 'sorry' or 'I forgive you'. You will learn all that from people who are doing that. If you hang around them long enough then you will start doing that. Then you bring it back into your own family. Then everybody starts doing that, if they did not do it before. And that is working in all these sections of the wheel.

So, I am talking of about the first state of being with your mom, and the things that come out of it. So if your mom was always stressed out then you will always be stressed out. If your mom was always afraid, then you are always going to be afraid. You have to be with people who are not like that. Then you change that part.

So, all these things are with the mom's situations, and maybe they are like that all their life, and maybe you are like that too, or maybe you get sick of it and you change, and you are not like that anymore. You do not like her, because she is like that. Many things come out of it – many different situations – depending on the individual. Some just accept and continue to be like that, some say: "no, I do not want this!" and they change.

They need to copy someone to do it differently but first they have to identify and realize, that they have that problem. You write a list of things you got from mom: lack of affection, lack of trust, stress, fear, anger and frustration. If there is one of these things, or a couple of these things then you are going to be like that, or you are going to struggle with those things, when you are growing up.

Insecurity, lack of determination or lack of strength, lack of protection and then you see if you have some of those qualities. If you do, you have to get a mom who can change that – by copying – and then you will create: Protection, strength, determination, security, willpower to overcome frustration and still win on top, anger to calmness, fear to being not afraid – warrior, stress to calmness, happy go lucky, living for the moment, trusting somebody and being able to be affectionate without fear or without conditions. You have to change these things.

These are the things that… you see… frustration, living for the moment, having faith that it will turn out properly or better than what it is, and insecurity to security. So what I am saying is, that if you have one of these things, then you need the opposite. Maybe you have some of these things but some are not there. Maybe you do not have all of them, maybe you have ten of them or seven or four of them, and then you look at the opposite side of what you need. For example if you lack affection then you need affection. These are maybe the traits that you have: lack of affection, lack of trust, stress, fear, anger, frustration, insecurity, lack of determination, lack of strength, lack of protection. So this is what you have, which is what you copied from your mom, probably because of the situation she was in at the time. Maybe she was a single parent, or was not happy in her relationship or whatever.

When you adopt a mom you need a mom, who has some of the following qualities; affection, trust, calmness, warrior, happiness, living for the moment, having faith things will change, security, determination, strength and protection. So those are the qualities you are looking for in a mom. And then you will copy those things. Then you change.

Grandparents

So the next section is grandparents: Roots or no roots. So you do not know where your people come from. You only know about Adam and Eve, and you know you were Vikings one time, but you do not really believe in Odin and all those things because you became Christian, but you are not really Christian either. So you are going around trying to find something to believe in.

These are the things that should be established in you by your grandparents. So you should be smudging with them, or going to church with them. Then all your life you know God is there, even as a teenager, even as an adult you will always have a grasp, that God is there in some form. So you have some faith developed and established, but if you had grandparents that did not do that, then you do not have that.

That is why you need your roots. If you do not have roots, you have lack of faith, lack of direction, you do not know where you are going, lack of reasoning – so you cannot figure it out – you just sit there being dumb. You cannot figure it out. Lack of reflection – when I say reflection, I mean realizing what you did wrong, or what other people did. Lack of heritage, lack of language, lack of identity and lack of pride come from not knowing your roots.

These are the roots. That is why you need the roots. Another thing the grandparents teach you is about nature, plants, animals, the weather, your environment – how to read it, how to pick roots and berries and preserve food, not to waste, to share, to be kind and thankful, and aware of yourself and of course love and respect. Then traditions, which are part of your identity are taught and then you also create traditions for yourself like Christmas, presents and birthdays etc.

Dad *(repeating for better understanding)*

Dad, where you feel secure, safe, you look up to him, you admire him, to be proud, you want to be like dad.

You start copying your dad. You do what he does, and you follow his interests. If he is hunting you will start shooting, if he is a carpenter you start helping him build houses and if he is a winemaker you start to learn, how to make wine. You have no choice, You have to work for him which is how you learn, skills, listening skills, how to comprehend or figure out problems, and you will learn a little more about money, budgeting, how to save and build things and then of course love – your dad loves you – and he is a pillar – somebody you look up to. He is strong and you feel secure.

If you have these teachings then you are able to get a job and you can just do whatever is required. It is not hard to pick up what you want to do, like shovel or hammer something or gardening and you just sit down and listen, because when you were a kid your dad made you listen and behave.

If your dad was not like that, and then you try to get a job, and you are not listening to your boss and you just say: "take this job and shove it" then you are fired and you do not even know, why you are fired. You do not even know, that you have an attitude. All those teachings come from your dad: discipline and respect.

Dad's Way of Expressing Love

Sometimes dads have a hard time expressing love in a healthy way, or expressing their pride in their children. They will say: try harder, you can do better, you can get a better grade. In most cases the dad cannot even reach those expectations, so what he is trying to say to the child is: "I want you to have a better life than me. I do not want you to be stuck doing what I am doing. I want you to be a doctor, a lawyer or a brain surgeon, so try harder. You can do better than a B+, you can get an A+."

So that is their way of encouraging their child. It is their way of saying: "I love you", "I am proud of you" and "try harder." Of course it is not understandable to the child. He feels the opposite. He feels that nothing he does is good enough for his dad.

What could happen if that is what you experienced, is that you become a perfectionist and nothing is good enough for you. Even though people comment on your good work and the quality of the work you do, you will always find faults with it. It will never match your expectations, because you do not have reasonable expectations. You are always striving to be better than what you are, because your dad was pushing you. Only the day when your dad says: "I am proud of you, you did a good job" only then you will stop being a perfectionist. Then you will accept your work, as good quality work and stop finding fault with it.

So we really need this healing and realization from our father and from our mother as well. This is another way of parents saying "I love you" to the child, without saying it directly.

And of course the child misinterprets this and thinks: my parents never really supported me or loved me. They always expected more than what I could do. Nothing was good enough for them. You get these resentful feelings and feelings of rejection. Then the outcome is that you will never do the work you were meant to do. You do not believe in yourself, or you lose faith in yourself, or you give up. The opposite could happen and you become a perfectionist.

These things can happen. So talking to your parents, having them express their love, gratitude and pride in you, will eliminate some of these walls that you created for yourself and change some of your negative belief systems. It will enhance your faith in yourself, the security within yourself, your ability to try things and your effort to accomplish things.

Honesty - Adult

Affection is important at a young age and then kicks back up when as an adult you want to hug and love – hug your wife and your kids – then affection feels good again. When you are teenager you are too busy messing around. You are not laying there holding your girlfriend or your baby. You are just making love and going out drinking or partying. When you are an adult you want to lay there holding your baby or wife, start being affectionate again.

Little kids want to always be hugged. They will come to you and they will sit on you, and you will hug them and they will like that hug for a while, and then they will get up and go play again. Then down the road they need to be re-energized and then they will come and need another hug. They want you to carry them. They like to be held and be close to you, because that is what they are craving, that is what they need at that time in their life.

Parents and Grandparents Should Support Your Dreams

Your parents and grandparents should be telling you to go for your dreams. Love is their common thing. They should encourage you to follow your dreams with love. If you want to be a fairy godmother, you may wear wings and a wand and sparkly stuff and you will dream. They all allow it. They make you feel safe to go for your dreams instead of always warning you not to do that. Instead of warning you not to do something, they should be encouraging you and supporting you and pushing you to do it.

They should not be jealous of you, especially your mom and dad. So no jealousy! They should not be restrictive, restraining or condemning. They should not be trying to put guilt or shame or frustration on their child. They should be doing the opposite.

The Right People to Adopt

There are qualities people need to have to be the right people to adopt. It does not matter if they are fat or skinny. Spanish or Italian as long as they have those qualities, they will be good healthy parents and good role models to copy. They can be from Spain or the Blood Reserve, they can be from Japan or wherever as long as they have these qualities, they will be good people to adopt.

Some families are just proper, and do not show affection too much. So if

you want a deeper understanding of affection, then you have to be around affectionate people. You cannot be around people who are like you. You are trying to get away from how you are, or how your own family structure is. You are trying to get into a nicer and happier family, with a mom or dad, who are not jealous or controlling or dictating or blaming. You are trying to get away from what you went through. You are trying to fix those things that got messed up with you, because of what they did to you.

You are trying to go and get another kind of mom with a different attitude, a different outlook on life, a different respect for herself and a different way of looking at life itself. You go hang around that person, and she will show you things, that you have never seen or felt before. That is what you need, not the same stuff you came from. That is the whole idea behind copying. That is the whole reason behind trying to find a mother figure or father figure. You do not want to choose some person just because they are a nicer person. They are not going to show you affection if they are from that same attitude, or that same way of being as you are.

If all your people are cold, then do not try to find somebody from that same area, because they are all the same. They are all going to do the same thing or feel the same way. If you are going to a country where there was bombing and war., do not expect those people to express themselves in a healthy way. They will express themselves with fear, frustration and anger, because that is what they went through for years. They got messed up because of the war. Maybe their mom, dad or brother died and never came home.

They are holding back their feelings and stresses and everything because they went through war but if you come to Canada there was no war here. You will get a totally different kind of people. You have to understand all that stuff and take all of that it into consideration when you adopt.

These are the qualities and these are the things you have to try to see in adoption. This is what adoption means. It is trying to fill in the things you did not get when you were growing up.

If you did not have a mentor, then you had nobody to talk to. You do not have skills of expressing yourself to your partner, your friends or to your family. You do not know how to express yourself, because you were never given that chance, or you were never around people who showed you how to express yourself. By being around people who know how to express themselves eventually you learn how to do that.

What you need to be around people who are able to express themselves in a healthy way, because if you do not have that, then you are not going to know, how to express yourself.

Then your relationship goes downhill, because you do not know how to talk to your partner about what is going wrong, or how to listen to your partner about what is going wrong. You do not know how to communicate with your sister. You do not know how to communicate with your mom. You do not know how to communicate with your friends and colleagues. You have a hard time communicating or understanding. It is all because when you were young, those things were not there. Once you learn to express yourself, then you begin to understand what the other person is trying to say. Then you become lighter and happier, more aware, more secure and focused. It should not have to come at a point where you are so stressed out, that you finally have to express yourself. It should just come out naturally.

If somebody asks you 'can you tell me how you felt about this experience?' you can just come out and say how you felt, instead of just being shocked, because you are the center of attention, and therefore just say anything that will make sense to that group, but not your deep feelings about it.

You will just say: "Oh, I think it was a very good workshop" instead of really elaborating on it and explaining how it made you feel. Just saying it openly and plainly instead of being stressed and freaked out, because you are in the spotlight, and people are listening for your opinion. You are scared to give the wrong opinion – instead of just being strong, and giving your own opinion, the right one.

This is really why you need people who express themselves in a healthy way. This is what will change in you, if you adopt expressive parents and grandparents and are around them. You could see a couple who have been happily married for 20 years in Denmark and they are really traditional and everything. You ask them if they will adopt you, and they say yes. They do not express themselves, so how can you ever learn to express yourself? But you fixed your wheel by adopting parents or grandparents. But they were not the right ones! This is why you need to know what you are looking for. Let's say you need a tire for your car, you need to know what kind of tire you need or you may not get the right tire.

How to be Adopted

You should know what you need, and you pray for these things. Adopted parents and grandparents should have certain qualities. Once you start having a relationship with them you should not be judging them. If it is a Spanish or Indian person and they eat guts or cow brain – you should not judge them. Do not compare them to your upbringing. Do not go to South America and start comparing them to Europe Europeans. You should be non-judgemental.

You may not be able to move in with them, or maybe in some cases you can. You should try to spend as much time with them as you can. It depends on the individual as to how much time they need to change. The best is to actually stay with them for a period of time. Then you get a chance to copy. You should stay with them at least a month as it takes a month to copy.

I think the best is to approach them and ask them: "Can you be my adopted parents?" Then you have to act like a child of your age and be around them, helping them, listening to them, asking them questions, copying them and helping them to preserve things for winter,. If you are learning to make wine, then you have to get the grapes and all. That is how you learn.

You live with them for a period of time, at least two weeks to a month. I do not know how long time it takes, but it should be an ongoing thing.

How you know if they are the right ones? You pray about it! You pray to the Creator to give you the right parents and tell the Creator the qualities you need in the right parents. Then you wait and when you see them you will feel it inside. You will feel it in your heart. You will know it. It is not something you think about – it is something you feel. You will feel it inside and you go with that. Not everybody is perfect, but you will see that the creator will guide you to the right ones.

Being Adopted

There has to be a sense of belonging. A guest is just a guest, but if you are adopted then the parents teach you, and they get after you, if you do not listen. They are concerned and they give you advice about your life. They are obligated to try to help you become a better person.

As a mentor, I am obligated to teach you. That is my role. But if you are a guest, I do not have to teach you anything. I just make sure you are full, and that you are okay. If you are a guest, I am not going to teach you why you need to pray, after we kill a deer. I will just say at this time we pray.

If you are adopted then I will teach you the importance of praying. I will show you how to pray after you kill a deer, or whatever, and you have to actually hunt and shoot a deer. There is a difference between being a guest and being adopted. The mentor has an obligation to teach and a responsibility towards the person they are adopting.

Why Society / Mentor

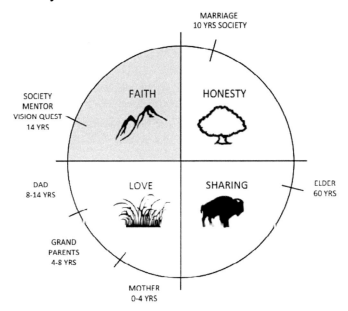

Some people are really outgoing, so they do not need the same tools as other people who are really shy and conservative. Everybody is different matter what culture you are in. You will have people who are quiet, people who cannot be quiet, people who listen and give advice, people who give advice but do not listen, outgoing people, people who sit in the back and try not to be noticed and people who try to fit in in a secretive or quiet way. Some people just come in unannounced. Every tribe, culture or nationality has people like that.

You can always see somebody when you understand the culture and you can see his behavior. It reminds you of your uncle or somebody down at the store. Everybody has these human characteristics.

You are Canadian and you just really like to talk a lot but your brother never talks. You find the same behavior in Denmark and Africa or wherever you go.

Some people do not have to work on society because they are outgoing, but actually a society is a really good thing to have for you as an individual. It makes you feel better, when you are with like-minded people with a common goal.

You get away from your family and your work for a little while. You have to balance your whole day and your whole life to be a secure person. You need certain qualities from your society. In order to learn to be safe with people, express yourself, talk, get along, share and come up with ideas and solutions and argue in a healthy way. You also learn people skills. That is what a society does for you. It also gives you a place to vent about things: Job or wife or kids or husband, the economy or no money or no job. You just vent and your society listens to you. It is like a healing circle. It is very important to have a society, because it eliminates frustration, and it also makes you feel that you are not the only person in the world going through something – other people are going through it as well, or are going through similar things.

It is just like thinking: "Oh, I do not have this!" – whatever it is. And you feel bad about it. "I should get this." Then you go to your society and there are a lot of people like you who do not have it either. Then it does not make you feel so bad, because you are not the only one even though you thought you were.

You find commonalities and then you figure out why you do not have it. There are a lot of reasons why you need a society.

You need to belong to something whether you are a mom or a dad, a sister, a brother or a grandpa. You need to belong to something, which is just for you. Something you like. You need your friends.

Maybe you have a friend or two but it is not the same. A society is a bunch of people doing something together. You are a brotherhood or a sisterhood. You back each other up. You are safe. You can express yourself. It is healthy. You belong. Maybe you do not have a husband a wife, kids, a girlfriend or a boyfriend and you are feeling bad about it. In the society there are other people who are in the same boat as you. There are other girls who do not have a boyfriend so you do not feel like you are the only one. There is a bunch of people like you or in the same situation as you so you do not feel like an outcast. You feel normal because there are other people like you. It gives you that sense of accepting yourself and gives your self-esteem and your security within yourself some stability. It makes you feel a lot stronger and happier. You are a happier person and that is important.

You have to understand that we all go through times of no jobs, deficits and this and that. You cannot get away from it but as long as you are happy going through all these situations… So, you can live in Denmark but you have to be happy. You can live in Africa but you have to be happy there. If you live in Mongolia you should be happy. Wherever you live is where you live but you should feel happy to live there. Societies help you feel happy and societies force you to look at yourself when you are not doing things right.

If you are really selfish your society friends can see it. Maybe you cannot see it. Maybe your wife is telling you but you are not listening because you never do. That is just the way it is. But when there are 12 members telling you the same thing you have to listen. You cannot say it is not true when all these people are telling you the same thing. Too many people are saying it is true so, you finally have to give in.

In a society you are able to see yourself. You are able to read people. You are able to understand things in a better way. More so than if you are just by yourself. If you are just by yourself – going through things – and somebody tells you: "I wish you would not talk about me!" That is just one person telling you that so maybe you will just think: "I do not like you anymore!" You do not see that person anymore but you never know that this is a problem with you. Later you make another friend and that person says something in a similar manner but you do not get it. You do not connect it to yourself. You do not think that you are being disrespectful. You just say: "I do not like you either!"

It happens to you three or four times and then finally you see a pattern for yourself or somebody tells you. You do not like it but you still do not change it. Later on you say: "well, I have been told that this is how I am. I do not think that I am like that but people say that."

You keep living like that or being like that, which can go on for years. But within a society when you say: "I am not like that." all these guys are saying: "Yes, you are!" You have to accept it because it is right there, right in front of you, right in your face and everybody is forcing you to see it. It is overwhelming and then you are finally forced to say "Okay that is how I am!" You change right there, and then instead of it taking ten years of people telling you that one by one. You do not like them or they do not talk about that with you, or they just put up with you. And you never change that. Maybe you finally accept that is how you are, but you still do not change it.

In a society you change right when the behavior is addressed. Then you become a healthier person earlier in life, so you and are more aware of yourself for a larger portion of your life. You do not want to do all this stuff at the last minute.

You want to do it now so you can realize what you are doing and correct yourself in order to be a healthier person. You are aware of your anger, and you know where it is coming from. You can take responsibility for it and get through it quicker. If you do not know why you are angry or where it came from you just take it out on people and lingers and you do not know why. There are a lot of people who do not have any help but when you are in a society, you have a lot of help. That is the reason why a society is really important.

When you have a mentor, you copy some things from him such as how he is or what kind of tool he is, his mannerism or just his outlook or how he does things, how he fixes things or how he sees things. You start learning how to do that. You start learning how to solve your own problems by seeing how he did it. You feel a sense of pride and security when you see that there is somebody taking care of you. So you feel worthy and of course there is that honor and that respect that you establish for your mentor. There is that discipline and self-discipline. You have somebody to copy, admire and respect. You have somebody to ask questions of, to feel safe with, you have somebody to lean on and ask for advice. You have someone to talk to about things. Maybe you cannot talk with your wife or your husband or your kids about it, things because they do not understand.

This is why we have these mentors. When life troubles you, go see them and they explain why you are feeling like this, or you are going through this, and how you can change it, and what you need to do. These are the things that a mentor can do. They can give you advice. You can choose to either take it, or not and use it to help yourself, or not do anything. That is your responsibility as a person. You get this sense of loyalty and protection. You start protecting your mentor because, he is protecting you.

You feel secure again because you have somebody who makes you feel secure. See all this is about feeling secure and safe because there are other things that are not there. Maybe you do not feel safe or secure with your wife or your husband, because they are screaming, getting drunk, or fighting, and you just get scared of them. Then you go to your society and you feel safe. Maybe they convince you to leave that person. You get help. They take care of you, they protect you, they stand up for you and they help you out. That is what members of the society should be doing – helping each other.

When you have your teacher, his or her job is to make sure that you learn. Sometimes they are nice and they talk to you. Sometimes they are strict with you, sometimes they get mad at you and sometimes they push you. They force you and they expect you to do something for yourself, and then you change. They encourage you. This is how we do things. This is like when I was sun dancing, and my teacher told us to jump in the river in the wintertime. He went first and then we all jumped in after him. This is the Indian way of mentoring. The teacher does it first.

You see that when I do healing Circles: I talk first and then everybody talks after me. Everybody is scared about who is going to talk first. Then somebody starts and it kind of sets the pace. Then it is easier. Some people do not have a clue how it works and after they hear it they go 'Oh, now I get it!' There is are a lot of reasons.

You are copying skills from the mentor to help yourself. You choose him or her because you see something in that person, that you need or that you would like to have. Let us say you want to be a good winemaker so you choose someone who makes good wine, and you go hang out with him and learn from him. Then sooner or later you learn how to make good wine. It might take a while but he teaches you how. Maybe you need to have patience and wait for a certain time and do some things, but at the end you know how to make it because he taught you.

There is a reason why you choose your mentor. It may be because there is an attribute in them that you would like for yourself. If he is outgoing and sure of himself you can learn how to be like that.

A mentor should lead by example. They should understand themselves, be open, honest, supportive, understanding, listen, give advice and they should be patient. A mentor should have all those qualities.

I live for the moment and feed my son pop sometimes. I just do whatever I think and whatever I feel in that moment, and I watch movies. But when it comes to sweat lodge and pipe ceremonies and Sundance, then I do it the proper way, the correct way, and I do it the old way. I got from my teacher that it is okay to be you – however you are.

I saw him for who he was away from ceremonies, and I saw him when he was in ceremony, and it was not the same person! This person was joking and talking about girls and stuff, and the next moment he is on the lecture talking about holy things, and everybody is really respecting him and admiring him, but nobody saw him joking the way he was, just half an hour ago.

He was being real! You cannot be a hundred percent holy. Nobody can. It is not possible. You need to experience all parts of yourself otherwise you are to go crazy.

It is just like some priests who do not have a wife, they do not have sexual intercourse with anybody, and the next thing is that they start molesting little boys in the schools and things like that. It is because they are not expressing that part of themselves. So if a priest was having sex with a wife or a concubine, then he is releasing that, and he is not going to molest those kids. When you restrict yourself then that part of you builds up. It is not good. You can turn into a serial killer or whatever. It could be a problem or a wall or whatever.

When you have a mentor you see them and you realize: "It is all right to be like this!" When I first became a Sundancer, I did not do anything bad. I never did anything wrong. I was just basically in spirituality all of the time, nothing else mattered. No friends or life! All I did was that.

I needed to have balance.

My teacher was saying: "You should with friends, go out a little bit, go to the show and enjoy yourself!" He was the one who got me to enjoy the other part of myself. I kept hearing spirits, and I kept hearing voices, and I kept hearing too much of it, and I told my teacher. He said that I was too much in that world. I needed to go enjoy myself and give it a break and give it a rest. I did not have to be working 24 hours a day. It was him who helped me to see that I need to have balance in my life between spirituality and having fun. Have a little fun – just being me.

During a period I was trying everything. I did not have a wife. Somebody would say: "try this!" and I would say "Sure, okay why not?" and then I was trying everything because I never tried it when I was a kid. So I checked it out and tried it out whatever it was. Now I do not need to wonder about what it would be like.

You should still be feeling okay with yourself after the experience, loving yourself and not feeling guilty or punishing yourself, feeling ashamed or embarrassed, or whatever you might feel like afterwards. It is just okay. That is another reason why you need a mentor.

Why Vision Quest

Before you go on a vision quest, you have to fix all the other things first. Or when you go up there you will only be fixing those things – instead of finding your purpose in life. You need to peel away those layers in order to get to your true self. When you have done that, you need to get someone to bring you up on the mountain. Someone who was successful and knows about it, someone who teaches you what to expect – and especially protects you. He also has to know ceremonies properly. In that way, you can get a good experience.

The vision quest comes after you have taken care of all these things.

When you go on the vision quest, you get this ability to see parts of yourself that you never see and other worlds that you have never experienced or seen. It is just like being in a dream. You go through different things, see different things and you come across different things. You may not know all of it, but you experienced something in a dream or on your vision quest. You may get confused or feel something, know something, see something or they tell you something. When you come down from the vision quest you get the messages interpreted, and then you know for sure, what it is all about. You know why you dreamt what you dreamt or why you saw a red cloth, or why there was a bear there. You get a real genuine explanation which guides you to what you need, the direction you need to go and what gift you have – whether you got a gift or not. It gives you something to go on.

There are a lot of people who do not deal with the things that I told them to deal with. They go on the hill and they do not get any messages. They are still stuck. I do not know how many people I bring up to Chief

Mountain because it is just the next step. They pledge and they are Sundancers and after four years then they go up there, because that is the next step. But all through their Sundancing they never dealt with their issues. After being a Sundancer, when they were preparing themselves to go on the hill, all they were worrying about, was their materials and their tobacco ties, and trying not to get angry. Then they go up on the hill and they get nothing, because of that certain issue, which they still have not dealt with all through their sun dancing. Maybe they are not even aware of that certain issue or they do not know why that could be a problem. There are a lot of different reasons or situations. It is like that. There are a lot of things that a society can do to help you.

All these things are helping you to feel safe, so when you go on the hill, you feel safe up there, and you feel accepted and wanted. Sometimes people do not feel accepted, wanted or desired.

There is this girl in jail who is really pretty, but she does not feel wanted. She knows she is pretty and she knows all these guys like her. She has to brush all these guys off, but she still has all these issues of being insecure and not feeling worthy. There is this other part of her that is aware that she is pretty, and she can get what she wants, but it is not enough. She wants to be accepted and wanted but not by the men or women. She wants to be accepted and wanted by her parents and grandparents.

She tried to find these feeling with her husband, but he had just copied the same problems that she came from. She is in jail because of drugs, killing, alcohol and all that. She expected to get this happiness from her boyfriend that she could not get from her mom. It was really false expectations and she still never got it. It does not matter who you are, or how you look. Every individual needs to feel loved and accepted by his or her parents.

A lot of people in this world have pain, because their mom told them they are ugly or no good or stupid, or their dad said those things. It sticks with them and they believe it. They do not try because they were told these things. No matter how they look, no matter how they are, they still have this personal deep pain that they got from their parents. These are all blockages that will stop you from finding your purpose in life, when you go on a vision quest. All these things can hinder the outcome of your awareness and then your vision – your purpose.

Some people do not go through all of this. They get a gift or they work through all these things, and then they go up on the hill and they get a gift. Some people know that they have to work through their issues but never did so when they went up there they got nothing.

Always in the back of their mind they think: "I wonder if it was because I did not do all this." You really have to fix all that stuff. Instead of wondering you should know why you do not get this and that. You know you need to fix this, and eventually you do.

Let us say that Saturday comes, and you have to get up. It takes you about half an hour to get out of bed. You do not feel there is anything to live for, you do not want to do anything, you are just bored or you are feeling lonely. You are just feeling bad about yourself.

So it takes you about half an hour to get out of bed and get going. When Monday comes along you still feel the same way but you will come out of bed quicker and get up and go, because you have a goal in the end. You have to go to work. You cannot just lay around and feel the world is on your shoulders, because you have to be at work. You get up and you go, because you have a goal. Saturday you did not have a goal, so why should I do this?

It is the same thing. Why do you need to fix things with your mom or your dad or have a mentor and all that? Why are you putting off doing it? Why you do not feel it is important or are too scared to get it?

So it is not that important. It is important but you take your time doing it. When there is a goal at the end of it all, then there is reason and that reason will carry you through. When you do not have a goal you do not feel like doing anything or you do not feel like trying, or you feel like giving up, or you have that miserable day, when you do not feel good about yourself.

You could say the reason, why you need to fix all this stuff is so, that you can go on your vision quest. It is the goal, and that will keep you going. No matter what happens this is the goal and that will keep you going. "Well, I need to change this, because I need to do that."

When you get your purpose in life, or something that you are supposed to do., then you get another apprentice or teacher to start working towards that goal. Maybe you are going to doctor people. You were shown herbs and how to doctor people so you apprentice with somebody, who is already doctoring people. You learn how to behave, how to doctor, when to rest, and doctor yourself and all that. That is another phase that you go through.

That is how it works. This is why you need those things to help you out, and find your purpose and follow it. Some people find it. Some people never do. Everybody does not have the same upbringing. Some people had grandparents, others did not. There are a lot of people out there who do not even know where to start, what to do or how to fix themselves. Now you start to see why it is so important.

It is hard trying to do something when you are by yourself. Some people think, that if they had a partner, they would feel happier and it would be easier to do this and that. But the thing is, that your partner actually stops you from doing these things. So it is better to do it before you get a partner. When you are all healthy, then you get a healthy partner who is not like your last one and does not have the same problems that you did. If you fix the things with your parents then when you have kids, you will not do the same things to them.

People just do not wait. They get a partner, and try to go to yoga or to a sweat lodge, and their partner is mad or jealous. The partner does not want to take care of the kids in that moment so then they cannot go or they have to go home quickly afterwards. If you have to do a Tree Ceremony then the person over here, who is single and just has a job and their own flat can do her Tree Ceremony next week. When does the mom who is sitting next to her have time to do her Tree Ceremony?

It is really important to understand that having responsibilities like a partner and kids is getting in the way of freedom. Okay, they do not want that freedom anymore and they want to have a family. Fine, but fix yourself before you have that family. You will be healthier and attract a healthy partner. That way you have a healthier family than by copying the family you came from, and doing the same thing to your daughter or your son,that happened to you.

The thing is that you are not the only one, who has those problems. There are so many people out there who have similar problems and probably even worse. Some people do not even know about the wheel and the steps, and they do not know they have to adopt parents or grandparents.

All they do is to wish they had a different mom or dad, and accept it. They grow up and have their kids, and do the same thing to their kids. They never had any awareness that they could fix it. They never had an opportunity to fix it. Now you can see the things that you need to fix, and the things you need do.

You know that you have some things to fix so you have no excuse. A guy who does not know what to do, has an excuse but somebody who has the tools and does not use them, has no excuse.

Adoption   The Qualities of Parents and Grandparents
(repeated for better understanding)

You have to look at the qualities of your parents and your grandparents. The things you were lacking from your mother are the things you want in your adopted mom. An adopted mom has to be attentive, secure, non-stressed, rooted, know her culture, raised properly or traditionally – knowing right and wrong, raised with attention and security herself, open minded, affectionate, verbal – what I mean by that is that she says: "I love you!" These attributes are what you are trying to copy.

Your adopted grandparents should know history, practice their culture and customs, understand beliefs, roots and original stories of their original people, their origin including where they come from, and how they were created, patience, and unconditional love,. They share stories, laugh, teach you things about life, and they are wise and loving. As long as they should have these attributes to copy.

Your dad has to be strong, honest, protective, loving, and affectionate and sets a good example. He is a teacher, a leader and a provider. He can fix problems, teaches by example and walks his talk: Humbleness and humility. As long as they have those attributes they are good parents to adopt.

Your parents and grandparents should be telling you to go for your dreams. Love is their common thing. They should encourage you to follow your dreams with love. If you want to be a fairy godmother, you may wear wings and a wand and sparkly stuff and you will dream. They all allow it. They make you feel safe to go for your dreams instead of always warning you not to do that. Instead of warning you not to do something, they should be encouraging you and supporting you and pushing you to do it.

They should not be jealous of you, especially your mom and dad. So no jealousy! They should not be restrictive, restraining or condemning. They should not be trying to put guilt or shame or frustration on their child. They should be doing the opposite.

Society

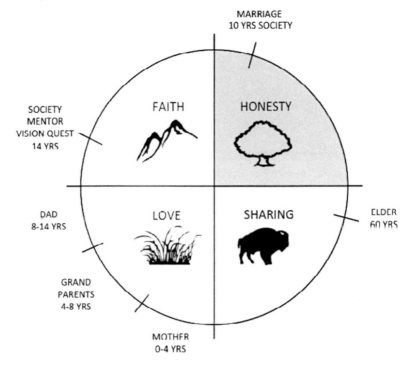

A society should have a society name, a society song, and society colors and then it should have rules, regulations, code of conduct, support, unity, goals and objectives. It must stand for something and be a protectors in some respect. Societies should be examples for each other and discipline their own members in private.

Long ago societies developed through dreams. People had dreams of different animals and these animals, gave these individuals a song and a way of dancing. It could even be from pigeons. The kid foxes created a society for people, and the buffalos created The Horn Society. The societies came from the animals. They felt sorry for us and helped us. So this is how these things originated.

In the process these people followed the spirit of the animal as well as animal. In these societies there is the leader, there is the second leader and then there are the members. In these societies all the members have clothes, headdresses or something resembling the animal that gave them that society. It may be a bunch of feathers, a rattle or a spear but everybody will have some symbol of where that society came from. Usually the members of a society were all around the same age.

These people had rules and regulations as to how to conduct themselves and how to behave within their society and towards the community. The societies had different purposes. Some were for protection of the camp and some were focusing on conflict resolution. Some were deciding where to move next – where the buffalo were.

The societies had different roles within the camp. They knew their roles and they followed them. If anybody broke the rules, the societies would punish them, but if their own members broke their own rules they were punished harder. The people saw that, and they saw that these people were not fooling around. They really punish their members if they make mistakes, so you had better not make this same mistake. It showed that they were fair. They did not favor their own members.

So let's say that you are in the police force. If a police officer does something wrong then the police force will back him up even though they all see that he did something wrong. They will protect one of their own. That makes people feel that if the police are not just. Why should they listen and follow the law when the police break the law?

So in the Indian way, when the people saw that the societies do not favor their own members, that the law is the law right across the board, then there was respect for the law, and for that society. People listened to the society without being forced to. There was no dictatorial stuff.

When there was a meeting about the camp each leader of each society would come to the meeting in the chief's house and then things would be decided. Then each leader would say: 'my society will take care of this' and the others said 'my society will take care of this'. Then they would go out and enforce the decision of the chief in council. It was really hard.

The people listened to the societies. It was the societies' responsibility to make sure the camp was protected, things were fair, justice was done or disputes were settled. Each clan had some members of the society living in their clan but when they came together as a whole Sundance where each clan members would come together and make the whole society group.

A clan is a group of Indians who live together. Maybe there are 200 of them. That is one clan and there is another clan that has maybe 150 members, and another one that has 80, and another has 300 members. These clans are all from the blood people as an example. They are all from the tribe, but they live in their family groups. They do not all travel together because it would be impossible to travel with 3000 Indians following the buffalo. These family groups spread out, so maybe you have 20 family groups that make up the Blood Tribe. These groups are called clans.

The tribe does not meet until there is a Sundance, and the whole camp comes together. In each clan there are members of each society. That is the only time when they can meet as a group – as a whole society. So for example if your membership for a society is 300 people then those 300 people will not meet together unless everybody is together. Each clan has some of those 300 members – maybe that clan has 10, that other clan has 20, and another clan has 30 members of this particular society. The members are all 30, and belong to this society, but they are in this little family group hunting in Banff, the other one is down in Cardston, and another one is up in Calgary.

These society members belong to different clans which are not together until they go to the Sundance and are a whole group again.

Once the whole group is together, then the societies come together, and the leaders say 'there is a lot of us, so no hunting until we decide who goes and who stays!' If the whole group goes hunting it will scare the buffalo and everybody will be hungry. Some individuals try to go hunt and they are stopped by the society, and they are disciplined. Another society will be watching the camp, at night so that nobody steals the horses. There is an older society which may be sitting there listening to two people having a fight and arguing about something. They are there to resolve it like court.

Each society has responsibilities in the camp. Some are police, and some are protectors. They had a role and a responsibility and a duty to the camp. In their own society, they had rules and regulations about how to behave and what to do, and they had systems. They met and they did rituals, they had dinners, smoking and storytelling. They did whatever they needed to do in their society to make it strong. They always had an older person who gave them advice. These societies have different age groups with different responsibilities.

Belonging to a society gives an individual a place to go. They have the same issues, and the same problems, because they are the same age. They are going through the same situations, so they have healing circles, and they talk about it. They share things, they talk about things, and they exchange ideas and values and understandings about life. They are educated there by the other members.

Maybe you never hunted and another guy did. He starts telling you about hunting, you discuss it, and now you know a little bit more. You had your friends, your meetings, your colors and your songs. You were busy, and you changed both your attitude and your behavior with everything that you learnt.

This is how it was, and this is what the societies' responsibility was. You belonged to the society and you did what the society said to do. Everybody decided what to do, and how to do it. Everybody agreed so that was the law. Every 5 years the society would move up to the older society, and they would give their society to a younger group. You had societies for 14 year-olds, for 17 year-olds and some for 20 and 25 year-olds etc. So every five years you moved up to the level of the next society and they moved up to the next level. You tried to be in every society throughout your life.

When they moved up the next society, whatever that society stood for, they took over that responsibility. When they were in a young society, they took care of hunting, and then they moved up to an older society which took care of disputes in the camp so they stopped hunting filled a new role. They took care of that responsibility whatever it was which was how it was in those days.

Today we do not have that same structure. Today we do not hunt buffalo, we do not have to protect the camp anymore, because we have police and courts that take care of all these things that the societies used to take care of. Societies used to look after things which the court, the police and the army now look after. This is why societies were there, and what they did for the community. Now we have all these other things in place, so it the structure is not going to be the same as it used to be. The roles and responsibilities of the societies change. You take the outlines of the structure and you implement them in a modern way.

There is police protection, okay, but you still walk around in the community and make sure that nobody breaks windows. If you see something, then you phone the police, and they come and get that guy.

That is the roles and responsibility of one society towards the community. An individual in a society is getting friendship, changing behaviors, new ideas, awareness and the ability to look at themselves in a different way. If you are by yourself, and somebody tells you that you have a problem you do not see that. Then somebody else will tell you the same thing, and then somebody else and somebody else... Maybe a year later you finally say, accept that you have a problem. You are not going to believe one person but if you hear the same thing from several people you have to believe it no matter how stubborn you are.

These things helped you with your character defects, prevented you from running away from yourself or other people and hiding in a corner. You had to show yourself, face what you were doing, and you had to change it. The main of the society in today's wheel is to force you to look at yourself. Your peers are making you do that, and because you belong to that group, you have obligations and rules and regulations in that group to follow. You have things to do. You have friends and you are active. You are a little bit happier, because you can be stress free. If you stay in a relationship all the time, and you do not go out and get away from that relationship, then you get into more fights, you get frustrated and maybe you break up. In a society you get away from your family for a while, you are with your friends, and you do other things. You can stay in that relationship longer because you have a break. That is what a society does.

You take the outlines of how they used to do things long ago, and you modernize it. We do not hunt buffalo anymore, and we do not protect ourselves from the enemy anymore. We go to the grocery store, the police protect us and the court decides about arguments and stuff. So you cannot take on the same structure they had in the 1800's, so you have to create your own rules and regulations today. The society decides what they have to be. I cannot say what you need to do. Every society is built for a different reason. I will be talking about Sundance, taking care of animals, Sundance and helping people with prayers and ceremony, so my idea of society is not going to fit in a society of librarians, who want to make a society because they are different. They read books, they do not Sundance. Whatever librarians need to do, to make their society work, is different than what I would do to make my society work for me, if I were a hunter or Sundancer or whatever. Other societies are not reading books, are not in the library and are doing different things, so that group of librarians needs to find their own rules and regulations, to fit their needs today.

A society needs an outline of the old days and modernize it, to fit their needs today. Get together and make your rules, have meetings and have something that your guys are going to be doing for the community. Everybody has input on the rules and regulations. People need to understand, why they need to be in a society, and how it will benefit them. Every group of people has a different view and a different way of thinking of how things should be, and they have to decide that within that group. Every society should have a responsibility towards the community. So for you as an individual... You have to have a reason to have your society together. You have to have projects and goals but you should do something for your community too.

In a society you have you have your colors, you have a society song, and you have rules and regulations. In a men's group or woman's group they do not have that. You have to take it a step further. In a society the members come wearing hats or shirts that say that they belong to this society. It is a totally different thing. Sundance is a society, we all wear skirts and medallions when we go there. You can see that that person is a Sundancer. In a men's group we all wear different clothes, we are not wearing any colors, and we just go there after work in our own clothes. It is just a group, it is nothing. There is a difference between a group and a society. In a group you do not wear colors

It is a Brotherhood. It is like a gang but a positive gang. Hells Angels all wear jackets, that say Hells Angels, but if you are going to the library to join a men's group, you are not wearing a jacket saying: Men's Group. There is a big difference between a group and a society.

Forgiveness

We are talking about forgiveness, the importance of forgiveness and some ways to forgive.

The importance of forgiveness is freedom from a hell that you create for yourself. When you do not forgive an individual that hurt you, you put a lot of negative energy towards that direction. What comes from that is the return of negative energy. What goes around comes around. You do not seem to have the good luck and good the synchronicity that you need in a job, relationships or attitude. Instead you have this bitterness, this anger, and this resentment that is like a stone.

That stone is blocking you from being free and experiencing happiness, goodness, trust and faith in people again. This rock is in the way so the energy does not flow, you are stagnant and this circular, negative energy seems to constantly come back to you. That is what it feels like. It takes energy to keep up that anger and resentment towards an individual, and over time it takes even more energy to keep that negative energy towards an individual.

"Time heals everything" we say, so the more time that passes in which you do not make amends with someone, the more energy it takes to maintain that resentment and that lack of forgiveness. You could use all this energy in other, more positive areas.

It stops the natural growth from continuing to occur for you to become wiser and see things from a different perspective. You are also robbing yourself of the opportunity to trust or to have faith in someone again, because you are denying that person, and yourself better possibilities, because you are not forgiving. So you are kind of living in your own personal hell, with of all these negative things happening. As a result you do not have too much good luck.

You put up walls so as not to let anybody in, which effects your emotions and your heart. You then become less sensitive in all these emotions that we have. Lack of sensitivity and the lack of ownership of your feelings happens because you are refusing to forgive, to learn and to relearn.

What happens when you do not forgive people and you do not forgive yourself at the same time, is that subconsciously you are not happy with yourself because you are doing something negative? The good part of you wants to forgive, but the rest of you are saying "no". Somewhere inside of you, you know better but you refuse to go there.

Forgiveness is a freedom that creates more trust, more bond and more strength in future relationships with people and it is not so fragile. You become wiser and stronger when you forgive. Too much pride makes a person weak, but they think they are being strong, if they do not say sorry or admit they are wrong. They think they are pretty strong but actually they are weak.

When you forgive someone, first you have to understand what they were thinking, or what the story behind their action, what they said or their behavior was. What was behind that? What caused that individual to act the way they did that hurt you? In some cases it may have been a repetition of behavior, a reoccurring thing. You look for the pattern and the reason behind it. The first part is to investigate and learn about the story behind the situation. You can ask them.

For example you might ask your mother what her relationship was like with grandma. Was she there? Was she affectionate? How did she treat you? How did you feel around her? Chances are that it might be the same as how you feel towards your mother.

If you do not want your children or future children to have the same kind of mom that you have, then you have to heal that situation with your mom or you have to adopt a mom. Otherwise your behavior will show up in your parenting skills. The pattern that you went through with your mother will repeat itself. You may not be aware of your behavior towards that child most of the time but maybe someday you will see, that you were exactly the way your mother was. That is not what we want.

We want healing. It is very important that you try to fix these situations with your parents, so you become a different parent to your children. What also happens is the opposite side of the spectrum: let us say that you were too disciplined and maybe you were spanked. You say that you will never spank your kids. You grow up and you remember what you said and you never spank your kids. The children grow up with no boundaries and no discipline. You are on the other end of the spectrum so the children grow up expecting things and not having to work for things. It is just as damaging to go to the other extreme of what you experienced. The middle is where you try to get to.

This is another reason why you need to forgive. If you understand the story you come across, by asking them about their life and their relationships with their parents, from there you can detect why they behave a certain way, or why they are this way or that way what comes after that is perhaps a discussion with your mother, about how she treated you, if you want to go there. You can just accept that this is how she is, because of the things she went through. Then you can say "I accept how she is" because of what she went through. Then the next step is to forgive. That comes naturally afterwards.

You also need to explain when she hurt you and how she hurt you. You need to get that off your chest, but you do not say that in an angry way or in a screaming way, but in a really kind, gentle way. Perhaps afterwards she explains things and her feelings towards her mother, Maybe she will be open to accept and realize that she is doing the same thing to you. Perhaps then healing can occur and then true forgiveness comes out of this situation.

The other thing you can do is to copy an adopted mom who has strength, love and affection. When you copy this you become like this adopted parent. You change your behavior through that adopted parent, and then the love and healing both come.

True Forgiveness

True forgiveness has to come through these steps that I just explained. Some people say "I have forgiven my mother" or "I have forgiven my father" but they are still angry, and they still have walls up. Perhaps they have forgiven their parents from the mind, but not from the heart. That is not true forgiveness.

You have to understand the story behind the situation and then you have to accept that this is the way they are, because of the way they grew up or whatever reason there is to the story. Then what naturally comes is the feeling that you have truly forgiven them. This takes time. If you do not know the story behind what they did and you say "I forgive you" it is not a complete forgiveness.

You will always have this distance from them and lack of love and affection, because nothing really changed. The relationship is still the same. When true forgiveness occurs, then the relationship changes for the better. There is more openness, love and trust.

Sometimes you cannot reach forgiveness with your mother. Perhaps it is not possible at the moment. That is why I keep saying that you should adopt a mother who you can learn these qualities you need from, so that you are not wasting years waiting to forgive, and waiting for your mom or dad to come around to talking about the feelings. Adopting a mother and learning from that mother will heal you quicker and you will change.

You are recopying, you are relearning to copy another way of being and so the immediate effect is that you copy your adopted mother: you open your heart, you learn to love and then you become a different mother to your children but you still need to forgive your own mother. Your ability to be a different parent has already been taken care of which is the immediate thing that has to happen. Then the forgiving of your mother can take its natural time.

If the parent is deceased, then you have to ask your aunt what your mother was like and how grandmother was to her. You can ask questions of some-one who knows the family well, or maybe your mother's friend, because maybe your mom confided in her best friend. There are many ways to find the story to help you go through this process to forgive your parents. But still I cannot emphasize enough that you get an adopted mother to copy. You cannot get around this. There is no way that you can change the way you behave, on your own. You are not going to get it from a self-help book. You need to copy somebody in order that receptors in the brain get reprogrammed. This is a critical thing to understand. If you want to change you need to copy somebody else who is the way you want to be. That is the way you change your behaviors.

If you want an open heart then you have to hang around people who have an open heart. Then you feel the feelings, and you learn to give the feelings back. If you do not express your emotions, then you have to be around somebody who does, and eventually you copy that, and you learn to express your emotions. Whether it is your mother, a friend, your boyfriend, adopted sister, adopted parents, or adopted family, you will learn to change eventually if you hang around this atmosphere long enough.

Addictions

If you did not get the attention, love and eye contact from your mother or whoever raised you, your brain did not develop properly. If your parent was stressed out and worrying all the time, then you become like that which is when addictions come. Alcohol or drugs enter the body and give you this feeling that you never had before of safety, of self-assurance, pride or feeling of love. People like that feeling, and these outside chemicals create this euphoria or that feeling that every human being needs. In order to fix addictions, you have to replace these feelings of love, affection and being wanted.

You look at somebody who lost his wife for an example. He does not have someone who loves him and he no longer has somebody else to love. It is gone. So that part of his affection is missing. To replace it or to forget about it, get over it or feel different, maybe he starts drinking and perhaps that becomes an addiction to take the place of the lost wife. They have to have closure with that relationship. They have to have a healing closure and say goodbye to their wife. Then your desolation, and the bad feelings are gone. Perhaps down the road they get remarried, so that emptiness is replaced. Then they do not need the alcohol.

Or as a child and you did not get the love, you needed and you grow up and you have addictions. If you replace those addictions with an adopted mom, or the things you did not have as a child, from an adopted mom, then there is no longer a need for the drugs or the alcohol because you are receiving what you need from outside now. It is all about feelings and love.

The Path of the Buffalo

Love, Faith, Honesty and Sharing

Love when you are born, how it is developed inside of you is what you are seeking as a human being. That is what you need at this time to grow and to connect. Your brain is developing outside the womb. Things in your brain that help you cope with life include happiness, joy and curiosity.

In order for a person to develop properly and be healthy all the chemicals in the brain and the connections require the child to receive love and affection.

The child's development also depends on how the mother is. The child is going to grow and feel things the same way the mother does. For example, if the mother is stressed then the child is going to be stressed growing up and it is probably going to take outside things to calm the stress down. They easily become dependent on outside things. It is because inside of them they did not develop properly.

The body always remembers all these things, and then the mind remembers after age 3. If the mother is not there with the child then the body remembers being abandoned by the mother even if she was only gone for a little while. Insecurity is created in that child if the mother is always going away.

That is why it is important that the mother is constantly with the child. The main caregiver could be the father or grandfather. – Whoever is raising the child from birth to 3 years of age has to constantly be with the child so the child does not feel abandoned.

The caregiver should constantly give eye contact and hugs and love and reassurances to the child and respond to the child's needs.

This helps the brain develop the things it needs to take care of itself down the road. The child then grows up to feel secure about himself and to love himself and to know that he is important and worthy. He is better able to say no to wrong things and everything functions properly.

It is love that helps develop the brain and the body from birth to three years of age. That is what the child needs. The child constantly wants to be hugged and sit on the mom and dad's lap and he needs a lot of hugs and embraces.

At four the child is able to talk and to comprehend and to copy. He can use the bathroom on his own. This is when it becomes the grandparent's responsibility to educate the child.

Then the child is with someone who lives for the moment, is very wise, teaches the child, and does activities with the child. The grandparent listens to what the child is saying, and teaches the child about his culture and roots. It is an introduction to his identity at a very young age. The grandparents are a major factor in the child's identity, who he is, where he comes from, who his relatives are and which clan is his. That is all done through love. The brain is still developing and the heart is learning to share and learning the reasons behind sharing, being accepting and friendly, kind and gentle, and learning to be happy instead of angry.

The grandparents help the child develop even further. Then when they are 8 years old, they are able to learn, comprehend and understand consequences. They go to school and an elder teaches them.

An example is archery: all the children are learning to shoot archery at 8 years of age and the ones who are very natural the elder does not spend time with. It is the ones that need a lot of help, who are weak and clumsy that the elder spends the most time with. The elder is trying to get them to be as good, as the natural ones.

After a lot of time and encouragement then these children begin becoming good at archery so that everybody is good at it. The ones who had to learn to be good at archery feel that they are like everybody else.

There are some that just cannot shoot, no matter how hard they try. The last resort is, that the elder or teacher gives the child his spiritual gift which is perhaps an arrowhead, and as he is gifted and noted for his archery skills. The elder gives the child some of his gift and now the child is better than everybody else. He does not look and he hits the target. He excels above anybody in archery, because he is gifted with something spiritual. As you can see nobody is left behind in this education. It can also be in running or whatever they are being taught.

The Path of the Buffalo

At the same time they admire their father and they want to be like their father. They start imitating their father as well as what he does for work. They listen to the father. He is their first hero, and how the father conducts himself becomes the child's belief system.

If the father is honest and straight, then the child picks up these ways of being, and respects them and tries to follow that same example. That is why it is very important for the father, to show the child a good example on conduct, self-esteem and belief systems. If the father believes in honesty, and the child listens to this then he makes it his identity and his belief system as well.

That is why love is so important in this first stage of development because it is helping the child to develop into a healthy person who is capable of showing love and receiving love in a healthy way.

He is not afraid of love and affection or afraid of people, but is happy to be with people because we need each other. We need to be held, we need to be loved we need to love we need to hold. This is human behavior. We are meant to live in communities, and we are meant to have a partner and we are meant to have children, and our bodies, mind and heart want that. There is a certain age when you want to have children as a man or as a woman. At that time it is only natural to have these feelings.

It is just the human part of us, the natural part of us to have children. Human beings are just like animals in the need to have babies to continue their species. and that is what human beings do too. We show love, attention and affection, and we ourselves try not to be stressed out or angry or afraid around the child so that the child, does not pick up on these feelings. We want them to learn in a very healthy way about the heart and not to be afraid of their feelings, or afraid of people and their feelings. This helps the brain to develop and everything to connect properly.

Then you become a teenager and in the teenage section or of time you are learning about faith. Faith in your abilities, faith in yourself and your thinking and what you decide, faith in the Creator, and faith in people: such as parents and teachers. You are learning to develop faith and trust in yourself.

You need some help and you need some guidance. As a teenager you start learning how to be social, have friends and to try to fit in, because that is what is important for them. After they have reached puberty it is good to put the teenager in a group of the same gender and the same age such as all 14 year old boys in one group and all 14 year old girls in another group. Because the hormones are all over the place you need a society to help balance these hormones and help the teenager into the next stage in life. What is important to him is that you accommodate that.

You put him into a group of people which we call it a society in the native way. They have common goals, common interests and they all have the same colors, maybe a shirt. They belong to a group. The people who belong to this group have rules and regulations as well as duties and responsibilities. They start to learn about loyalty and brotherhood or sisterhood. They support and help each other, they learn to be social at this time, to get along with people, and how to speak to people properly. By belonging to a society they have things to do every day start to learn about responsibilities, which help in developing the faith part.

Next thing that comes is challenging other societies. You learn to be devoted to your society and back each other up, and then you know what loyalty is. Then you learn support, and because you challenge other societies, you try to maintain good members within your society, so the other societies do not find faults in you and tease you, or make fun of you or your society, If you are not behaving properly your society members will come to you and address this issue with you. Because you want to stay in your society and in your group, and you do not want to be ostracized you change your behavior, which is for the betterment of the group, and the betterment of yourself and your family and the community as a whole. The societies discipline each other and encourage each other to be better human beings. You challenge other societies which is entertainment for the camp or the community.

Another thing to do is to get the teenager a mentor, because the teenager is learning about faith and learning to be a little bit more independent. Sometimes they are too close to the parents, so they do not respect the parent or listen to what the parents say about things. If the teenager has a mentor whom he looks up to, the teenager would listen to whatever the mentor would tell him.

It has nothing to do with parenting skills, teenagers are just like this. It is through the mentor that the parents get the message to the teenager whether it be doing their homework, trying harder in school or cleaning their room or maybe behaving more appropriately.

The parents will discuss this with the mentor, and then he will find a way to talk to the teenager about this behavior, without pointing fingers at the teenager. Perhaps the mentor will use himself as an example, and tell a story from when he was that age, about what he did and what he learned. The teenager does not have to feel threatened, because that he is getting a lecture or something. He is listening to somebody's story, and because he wants to be so much like his mentor, he copies the positive things in the story such as trying harder in school. He is copying the positive things.

At the same time the teenager is growing up, and is experiencing things, trying things, and having results from these things which he wants to talk about. Maybe he met a girl and he is feeling something for the first time, and he does not understand the feelings, or how to be with a girl properly. He wants to ask questions and needs some guidance.

A mentor is a little bit more open minded than a parent. If the teenager is in trouble and needs to talk about this problem he talks to the mentor, and then the mentor gives him advice about what he should do. If the teenager went to the parents and asked for the same they would probably give him a lecture, because the parents are too close to the child. The parents will not be optimistic or open with the child, or might give the child a lecture or tell him that he should not go out with girls at such a young age.

The teenager is not going to feel safe talking about his feelings with the parents, because of the anticipation that he is going get in trouble, or get a lecture. With a mentor he will feel safe, and less apprehensive about sharing openly and honestly. Sharing is a natural feeling, that human beings experience at an early age.

Then, of course, it is also about faith and finding yourself and finding your purpose in life. So the last thing you do for the child, is to put him on a hill for a vision quest to go find his purpose in life. So the teenager is given a pipe and goes on a hill with a buffalo robe, and he spends four days alone without food or water seeking his purpose in life.

Because he is young and does not have many layers of scars: emotional scars, spiritual scars and mental scars, it is easy for him to connect to his soul or his spirit. That is where the answer is to what his purpose is. He might get a dream or he might get directions. When he comes down he tells the medicine man about what he experienced, and the medicine man will interpret his experience and from there, they can determine what he is supposed to be. It could be a healer, a craftsman, a chief, a hunter or artist. Whatever the child is supposed to be, will be revealed and then they put the child under an apprentice who is already doing that.

Maybe they find out that teenager will be an artist, so they put him under an apprenticeship of an artist. Another one is destined to be a craftsman and he is put with a craftsman. They can understand each other and the way they feel towards their art.

This is what the teenager goes through, when the faith is developed properly. The teenager is under the apprentice developing the skills of whatever he is supposed to be until he becomes an adult.

As an adult, honesty becomes important to the individual. He understands that honesty is important, and he starts practicing it himself. He looks for it in his partner, he looks for it in his friends, and he looks for it in his parents and in the government. At the same time he meets someone, gets married and starts a family. He is not used to living with somebody other than his parents and brothers and sisters.

Married couples sometimes need a break from each other and so societies are really crucial at this time. Societies provide them with a break from the dynamics of being married to another person and trying to be compatible.

Being with their own kind gives them a chance to talk about things that interest them like archery, weapons or sports and for the women they might talk about clothing, children or herbs or whatever is interesting to this group of women. They have a break from their partner and their family, and they get to be with people of the same age and same gender. This is to reenergize them so when they come back from this group and the activities, they are happy and fresh and they are better husbands and better fathers, better mothers and better wives, and better teenagers and better sons and daughters. These societies are so critical at this time to keep the family unit together and healthy and happy.

You are acquiring wealth at this time and a home. After ten years your wife becomes your best friend. You have lived with each other for ten years. You confide in your wife more than your friends now. Things change. You and your wife decide to join a society together, and there are other married couples with children that have been together for ten years. When you join a society together, it is usually a sacred society, so you have spiritual obligations. Perhaps you get a spiritual object that you have to take care of, and then the wife has to give smudge and the husband has to do sweats, You have a certain way of living now, and you bring your children up in a holy way.

This sacred object and the teaching behind it are about truth and honesty, and how to be a better person as an adult your age. So now you and your wife are taking care of the people through your spiritual walk.

You are being taught that you will never be as strong as you can be, unless you have a partner, whether you are a man or a woman. If you are giving energy to help people you are drained. When you come back home your husband or wife reenergize you and clears what you picked up, by holding you and being intimate with you. They do not pick up anything. It is just healed and reenergized through love and the affections of love. This is how the couples support each other through this time: spiritually, emotionally, mentally and physically.

You live this kind of life trying to be a better person and bringing your children up in a holy way.

Then you change again, as you become an elder. Around 60 you stop being in these societies. Now that you are in the old age stage you are compelled to share your knowledge about life. Now you are up early in the morning, teaching your 4-year-old things you learned from your grandparents about animals and identities, and plants and people and events, and stories about your history and people who made mistakes, and how mistakes were corrected through these stories.

Then you go to help teenagers, maybe as a mentor or by putting someone on the mountain. You may be a big brother to a society and you are helping the teenagers to go through the experiences they have to go through to develop themselves in a healthy way.

Perhaps you are a teacher for the children in school, maybe you are teaching the archery, horsemanship, running or hunting programs. You may be helping the adults with their sacred society, and giving them guidance, support and reassurance and running their ceremonies. You and your wife go and assist in this way.

This goes on until you are 80. By then you are getting old and tired and you are forgetting. Then you retire and you give the responsibilities of your job as an elder to younger elders to take over, and then you enjoy the rest of your years. Maybe you come to a ceremony for a little while, and then you get tired and you go home. Maybe you go to a society dance like a powwow, and you are there for a little while enjoying it, but then you get tired, and you want to go home early. You slow down.

Sometimes these elders make the end of their circle, and then they start again and become children again. They need a diaper, they need to be hugged again, they to be held, they repeat themselves.

Never feel sorry for these elders, but admire them because they completed their circle and they will not come back in human form. They will come back as spirit helpers, but not to try their wheel again.

Some people who do not finish their wheel properly will probably have to come back and try again to find their purpose in another life.

We all try to reach this circle and to complete it in this life time, and that is why we try to follow this wheel which was set up by our ancestors thousands of years ago, as a way of attaining a full healthy life in the circle of life. This is why each section is important, and what they are feeling in each of these sections: Love, faith, honesty and the last one, sharing.

Stereotypes

In this part I talk about different people, and what will be strong and what will be weak in these people. Be aware that I am stereotyping. Some people are not like this, but it is just to give an example of how some people might be. I am going to stereotype a little bit.

An individual who will be strong spiritually and mentally, and perhaps weak emotionally and physically, might be somebody like a priest or a monk. It is their vocation to be spiritual and then they are also very smart mentally, because it develops the psychological part in you.

But perhaps they do not have a partner or children, so they will never understand the full emotions about having a wife and children. If they are not very active because of their lifestyle, so the physical part may be lacking.

A choir singer might be strong spiritually and emotionally but perhaps mentally they are not as keen or sharp with mathematics or physics. Maybe they are bit scared of making decisions about life, and maybe they do not have the confidence, so physically they might not be taking care of themselves.

A scientist may be strong mentally but perhaps he is not very strong spiritually and maybe emotionally he is not giving the time that he needs to his family, because he is always busy, and maybe he is not taking care of himself properly. A doctor, psychologist or maybe an overworked lawyer might be the same.

You have other people who are very strong emotionally and physically like actors who know how to control their feelings, and need to have good bodies, or models that believe in themselves and love themselves in a way, but perhaps they are weak spiritually and mentally.

Football players and others in sports perhaps they are like this as well.

Some people are very strong mentally and physically. Perhaps they are really good in business and they exercise and eat well, but they do not pray as much as they should Maybe they are not really in tune with their emotions, like businessmen or doctors or somebody who works with his mind a lot but has not opened his heart and does not really pray.

These are different types of people and I am stereotyping them of course. Mind you, not everybody in these fields is like that. They may have connected with their heart and emotions, and maybe they are developing themselves properly, but others do not and they fall into these categories.

Supporting Dreams

Your parents and grandparents should be supporting you through love and encouraging you. It is healthy for a child to play out his fantasies whether it is by stomping around like a dinosaur or pretending to be a fairy godmother or a princess. Allowing the child to play out the fantasies without restrictions or being put down assists them in dreaming. Sometimes we buy them princess clothes or a dinosaur shirt, and we encourage them to act out and play out their fantasies and roles.

It gives them dreams and desires for the future. As they grow up they have an Idea of whether they want to become this or they are better at that. They may want to experiment or do try something different.

Because they had support and encouragement as children, they feel safe to try out that new experience, without allowing their fears to hold them back. They believe in themselves, so they go for that change or that goal or that experience later in life.

That is why it is so important as the child is growing up, that the parents and the grandparents really support them, and encourage them to fantasize, to play and to dream. That is where dreams come from, and how they develop and create, so that further down the road when you are older, you have these dreams and desires which are not impossible. They become possible.

You have to support your children and encourage them to be what they want to be no matter what their dreams are. (If they change their mind later) it is still their own responsibility to become aware of it if it is not good for them and change. All you can do is support them and their dreams and what they want to do...

If a Child Does Not Forgive

The only thing you can do as a parent, is to say I am sorry for what I have done, and try to make amends for it. If the child still does not accept this, there is really not much you can do, other than to say sorry. You have done your part. It hurts if the child does not accept it, but you have done what you can. It is up to the child to accept it or not.

One Section Back

If you do not fix your wheel then your maturity is one section back. You lack all this confidence and this awareness and reassurance of yourself that help you develop into who you are – who you should be.

You may be an elder but you do not want to take the responsibility of teaching your grandchildren or teaching others. Maybe you do not feel worthy of being such a person, or maybe you think that someone with more capability should do it instead of you.

All these factors show up; you do not feel worthy of being an elder or a teacher or a mentor. There is that lack of trust within you, that lack of ability, that not wanting to do it. Maybe you do not want to take on the responsibility. You are still thinking like an adult rather than an elder because you have not attained these things that give you the maturity in your heart and in your mind to act your age.

In the adult stage, there are 30 year-olds, or 40-year-olds, that cannot keep a partner. They go out on weekends trying to find a partner which is something that a teenager does, not somebody who is 30 or 40 years old. They should have outgrown the partying at that maturity level. They should have a partner, and be well into living together, have a family, a house and material possessions. Instead you have all these people, who cannot find the right partner. They go out on weekends and get drunk, and try to find the right partner, or they go on all these dating websites. They are acting much younger than what their age is.

Then you have teenagers who are troubled, and have lots of problems. When you start working with them and peeling away all these layers, what you find on the bottom of everything is that they just need to be loved, and to be hugged which was something that should have be done when they were children but they are still crying out for that. They are older and they should be working on other things like their faith and leaving the nest and getting ahead.

Instead they are troubled and have turmoil in their life because of the lack of love. Their maturity level is one section back, even though their physical age is that of a teenager. This is what happens when you lack these things.

The child is not getting all the things he needs and so therefore he is losing awareness. The roots are not established properly so they do not have the confidence, the ability or the freedom to grow properly, or the affection or the awareness or the constant attention they need to develop properly. This is what happens when you do not have all these things in place.

Stress and Addictions

When you are in your mother's womb and she is stressed out, or when you are born and she is in a stressful time in her life, you as a child will pick up on that stress when breastfeeding, you cannot help but pick it up.

Stress from your mother does not allow certain connections in the brain to connect properly, therefore when you grow up you will not be able to deal with stress properly. You are more susceptible to being addicted to something because you get stressed out easily.

What you can do to fix that problem, is that you copy or hang around people who are not stressed out, and eventually you start to copy them and you start being less stressed out.

You see it all the time. You see somebody from a big city who has a really stressful life, and then they travel to the jungle in South America. The first couple of days they will be adjusting to the different environment, the different energy and to the people who are not in a hurry, but are taking their time. The person will have to take a little time in order to adjust to this, and once they are adjusted to this new energy and the people, then they start to copy their behavior and to calm down and relax.

It is natural to copy the people you are around. If you are a really relaxed person, and you go to a place that is really busy. It is going to affect you. It is not going to be comfortable for you, and you are not going to feel good about it. If you are there long enough, you will end up like the other people, running around, rushing and stressed out.

You copy the people that you are around, whether they are good or bad. Eventually you will copy them, and you are not even aware that this is happening. It is a natural thing that occurs. When you around other people you start to copy them.

The brain does not know to release the things you need to calm down when you are stressed, because this process was not developed due to the fact that you were always stressed, because your mother was stressed. It takes time for this to develop, connect and heal. You need to be around people who are not stressed, and eventually your brain will create this state, and you will be able to take care of yourself and deal with stress in a good way.

Before this happens, you find it really difficult to deal with stress and you cannot cope with it properly. Maybe you have a drink of alcohol and it calms you down, and then pretty soon you drink a little bit more and a little bit more, and pretty soon it becomes a problem. Maybe you take drugs or medication from the doctor, or other things to relieve stress and then if you are not careful, you can become addicted.

The natural way of dealing with stress is to reprogram yourself and be able to deal with stress without having outside influences to calm you down. You should be able to calm yourself down. The brain is able to fix that. Once you are around somebody who is not stressed out, you will eventually start copying that, and then the brain starts fixing itself. You do not need outside Influence to calm yourself down, down the road.

Dependency and Grown Up Societies

In the past they had these societies. The man belonged to a society and the women woman belonged to a society. When they got married the societies celebrated their member getting married, and it was a big deal. You continued to belong to these societies. As a young couple getting to know each other, it was always important that you went to your society to have a break from married life. Marriage was new and exciting but also demanding, because you had to accept your partner's behavior and lifestyle, and try to make everything fit together. There is a lot of give and take in the beginning of a relationship as well as changing habits and patterns so everybody can coexist in a healthy way.

Today what you have is individuals coming together, and being in this honeymoon state, where they cannot stay away from each other. They hang on to each other and cling to each other. Sometimes this continues without a break or without seeing friends. Without having a society to go to, you do not have a break from each other. Then you start depending on your partner for your happiness. Nothing else matters than being with your partner.

If they do not have a break, from each other the stronger character may get bored, or they may both get bored of each other. One partner may get tired and the other one clings on. Then a very bad separation begins. They separate and come back to each other and that pattern repeats. Eventually they separate with bitter feelings or unsettled feelings, which create walls for future possible healthy relationships. It creates patterns where you find a similar person or similar characteristics in a new partner because of unresolved issues or unresolved closures.

So this is what you have today. When couples had societies, then they had a chance to get away from their partner, and have a break for a couple of hours with people of the same gender, the same way of looking at life, the same behavior and with the same interests. Then when you come back to your partner there is a happiness and revitalization in your thoughts and your feelings towards them and you feel more obligated to be a good partner. That is what societies really help with in the first ten year of the relationship.

Eventually you and your partner become best friends, and you do not confide in your friends as much as you used to. Now you start confiding and trusting more in your partner and talking with them about more things. After ten years your partner becomes your best friend and your childhood friends come second.

Then there is a state of maturity and realization and you want to do better for your kids, so you join a society together as a couple. This is usually by the pipe where you choose to live together forever. You get a bundle and then you start living the way of that society as a couple. There are probably a lot of obligations with the bundle. You take on the male role and your wife takes on the female role of that society. It takes a male and a female for these obligations to be fulfilled, so you need a partner in order to make these ceremonies which are designed for a couple take place.

After four years there is a transfer of the bundle, and some couples join another sacred society or get another pipe and continue that way of life until they are around 60. Then you become a grandfather or a grandmother, and you begin to share your knowledge. You feel compelled to share your knowledge with people. Then the work really begins because you now have to go pick up your four-year-old grandchild and begin to teach them about their roots. Then you go talk to the teenagers, you run society sweats or teachings for the society you and your wife belonged to. Your obligations become more when you are an elder. You have to take care of everybody, and you do this until you are about 80. Until then you are being depended on for speeches, prayers, sweats, teachings, guidance, advice, support, love and then around 80 you get too tired and you retire.

Talking to Parents and Forgiving

One of the obstacles about talking to mom and dad is, that sometimes they might not want to share or talk about certain things with you. So if you approach them with a question like "I was hurt because you did not show me affection" they might get offensive and they might shut down. Maybe that is not the best approach in dealing with fixing your wheel with your parents. Knowing how the wheel works is that you copy your parents, you copy their behavior and what they do and how they parent as well. You also copy grandparents and other people as to how to behave in society. Without knowing how to copy somebody we would not know how to behave in society or how to survive with each other. We copy each other whether it is regarding fashion, gestures, sayings or activities. We copy certain individuals. Some people go to operas, some people go to movie shows, and some people go to Bingo.

Probably the best way to approach your parents - knowing about the copying method on the wheel, you ask them: "Mom, how did you grow up. How was it with grandma? How did she treat you? What was your earliest recollection? Was there a lot of love involved or affection from your mom? What did you remember from her?" Then she will tell you a story and perhaps if she gets right into it, she will start talking about the things that bothered her, naturally to get it off her chest.

From this story you can understand why she is the way she is.

And then - knowing the wheel - you can understand that she copied it her behavior from her mother, that is why she is the way she is. Then you can accept her the way she is because of her past, her history, you understand it. Now it is easier to accept your mother the way she is, and what will follow from that is forgiveness. So at the same time you are giving her an opportunity to heal. Your mother may not recognize the opportunity to heal at that time or at the moment. That is one way you can get the story from her on how things were with her. You can see the pattern of her coping, and if how she was with you was nicer or perhaps the same as how she was treated or maybe not as extreme. You can be thankful about those kinds of things you see. There is a little bit of development from your mother towards you as compared to her mother towards her. So this is one method you can use to approach your mother.

It is helpful to understand your parents and then you can accept them and then forgive them. You can do that with grandparents as well. That is one way of opening the door to understanding, and perhaps further down the road, with more talking with your parents in this way you can slowly discuss what you remember in a non-threatening manner. It gives them an opportunity to see how you feel and then perhaps from that point in time there could be healing.

The thing is that once there has been forgiveness between the parents and the child, your behavior with your spouse will change overnight. Your spouse might feel like she has a different person in front of her which may also cause complications.

For example, maybe you were always arguing with your partner and when you fixed things with your parents all of a sudden, overnight, you are no longer arguing. Your wife is used to you arguing but you do not want to argue anymore. That creates a problem with your wife's attitude, maybe not consciously but subconsciously. She is behaving badly and you are not so she might feel less than you and expect you to argue back.

That might cause a problem which is why I encourage couples to attend or to understand the wheel together so that they understand the change and adjust to it. If only one spouse knows about the wheel and changes, and the other spouse is not prepared for the change it could cause problems between the two of them, even if the change is a positive one.

It is recommended that both spouses know about the change that can occur and try to adjust to it so that when the change happens, they both see the change, understand it and adjust to it.

If one partner changes it might make the other partner want to fix their wheel with their parents so as to undergo the same change that their partner did instead of separating, because you act differently than one another. One partner gets the "you do not argue with me anymore and you are too good so I will leave you" – attitude or decides that you are arguing and I do not want to so I will leave you. Instead of that happening maybe the partner can fix her wheel with her mom so they are both at the same level again. This wheel is meant to fix everybody and anybody in and around the person who is looking at it, because people get curious and want to learn how to fix themselves by seeing an example in front of them. These are the things that I think you have to watch out for in changing your wheel. Change can happen so drastically and you could change so completely, that it is hard to for people around you to adjust to that change overnight. You have to take that into consideration when you fix your wheel, because that does happen.

If you were arguing with your partner which you usually do and all of a sudden your partner stops arguing back you are like, what is this? The other person does not want to argue. You are not happy about this change because you still want to argue even though the other person does not. He is just happy. Everything is okay. It is not a problem anymore.

This will create something inside of you, because now you feel less than your partner, because he does not want to argue. You feel mad at them because you feel less than them in yourself. You take it out on them and you try to find something that they are at fault with or where they made a mistake. You will not admire the change, you will look for something that will piss them off instead of appreciating the change, because you have not changed.

This is a problem that the partner should be aware of regarding what the wheel does for an individual to change. If they know all about the wheel and they see this person change, then they know the process and then in-stead of being upset and trying to look for a fault in that person, perhaps it would encourage that person to try to fix their own wheel with their parents using their partner's method. Perhaps if they both fix their wheel they stop arguing, and they both have a healthier existence with each other. It is not just one person fixing their wheel so that they are not compatible and they separate.

It should be a continuation where the partner gets this energy, copies it, uses it for himself and his parents and changes as well. Now they are both at another level where they do not argue with each other. There is healing and then they have a better coexistence and a happier and longer life together.

Preview - Sequel

Coming soon ...

Camille Pablo Russell

"Path of the Buffalo - Medicine Wheel - Part II"

My next book is already in preparation and will be published soon. It will focus on "awareness":

Now that you have read this book– hopefully – you are now ready to fix your own medicine wheel, as you have learned about healing the bridges of your shortcomings. Now we can continue working with the tools of the Medicine Wheel.

I would like to deepen the focus on awareness of what God tells you and what your own spirit tells you. It's about intuition and survival, speaking in maturity is the moral of the story.

Listen to what the elder(s) is/are telling you. Open up your mind as a vulnerable human being. Grandpa will tell you the Napi stories, about how to do things, and how to understand the difference between imagination and projection. (About humbleness and humility? About forgiveness and unconditional love?) You will learn how to tell the difference between what God is telling you and what your own spirit is telling you and about how to feel secure.

Your mom, your grandparents and your dad will support you by telling you their stories, not just explaining, but also by supporting your intuition and making you feel secure.

Part II will give you the tools – the mental, spiritual, emotional and physical tools to walk your authentic and balanced path. Path of the Buffalo enables you to contribute your skills to your family, community, professional environment and society.

Contact & Credits

Copyright
Camille Pablo Russell - October, 2016 - Fifth Edition

Website
www.pablorussell.com

Transcript & Proof
Marlena Reimer Pedersen
Christine Doederlein
Martina Moser
Kjell Laursen

Photography
Jannie Nikola
www.nikola.dk

Cover
Kjell Laursen

First Edition Printed in Denmark
Trykteam, Svendborg

First Edition Publisher
ETNA Edition

Fifth Edition Printed in Canada
Friesens, Altona

Fifth Edition Publisher
Colouring it Forward

ISBN
978-0-9952852-1-7

Please visit the website: www.pablorussell.com for more information about Camille Pablo Russell. Here you will also find contacts for each country, and information about activities, and how and where to buy this book.